Adrian Baum

EVALUATION IN A
NUTSHELL

2ND
EDITION

A practical guide to the evaluation
of health promotion programs

  Medical

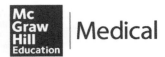

Medical

This second edition published 2014
First edition published 2006

Copyright © 2014 McGraw-Hill Education (Australia) Pty Ltd
Additional owners of copyright are acknowledged in on-page credits

National Library of Australia Cataloguing-in-Publication Data
Author: Bauman, Adrian E. (Adrian Ernest), author.
Title: Evaluation in a nutshell: a practical guide to the evaluation of health promotion programs/Adrian Bauman &
                 Don Nutbeam.
Edition: 2nd edition
ISBN: 9780071016209 (paperback)
Notes: Includes bibliographical references and index.
Subjects: Health promotion.
                 Health planning.
Other Authors/
  Contributors: Nutbeam, Don, author.
Dewey Number: 613

Published in Australia by
McGraw-Hill Education (Australia) Pty Ltd
Level 2, 82 Waterloo Road, North Ryde NSW 2113
Associate publisher: Sarah Long
Production editor: Lindsey Langston
Permissions editor: Haidi Bernhardt
Copy editor: Katy McDevitt
Illustrator: Alan Laver, Shelly Communications
Proofreader: Mary-Jo O'Rourke
Indexer: Shelley Barons
Design coordinator: Dominic Giustarini
Cover design: Simon Rattray and Dominic Giustarini
Internal design: Simon Rattray
Typeset in ITC Giovanni Std 9pt by diacriTech, India
Printed in Australia by Griffin Digital

contents

List of tables and figures   vi
About the authors   ix
Preface   xi
Introduction   xiii

CHAPTER 1

Planning for evaluation   1

1.1   Problem definition: starting at the end   3
1.2   Planning a solution   3
1.3   Creating the right conditions for the successful
      implementation of programs   5
1.4   Planning for the implementation of health promotion
      projects and programs   6
1.5   Health promotion actions and outcomes   7
1.6   Evaluation   11
1.7   Summary   13
References   16
Further reading   16

CHAPTER 2

Research and evaluation in health promotion: key stages, methods and types   17

2.1   Evaluation methods and types   17
2.2   Balancing scientific design with practical need   19
2.3   Stages of evaluation   22
2.4   Quantitative and qualitative methods in program
      evaluation   32
2.5   Formative, process and outcome evaluations   35
2.6   Summary   36
References   37

CHAPTER 3

Formative evaluation   38

3.1   Formative evaluation: testing methods and materials before
      starting a project or program of work   38
3.2   Formative evaluation for different types of health promotion
      intervention   47
3.3   Summary   48
References   48

CHAPTER 4

Process evaluation   51

4.1   Assessing the implementation of health promotion
      projects and programs   51
4.2   Methods for conducting process evaluation   54
4.3   Summary   61
References   61

CHAPTER 5

Evaluation methods for health promotion projects
(interventions)   64

5.1   Evaluation designs for health promotion projects   65
5.2   Selection bias and sampling   74
5.3   Statistical significance and data analysis   77
5.4   Health promotion measurement   79
5.5   Summary   87
References   87

CHAPTER 6

Complex program evaluation   89

6.1   Background to complex program evaluation (CPE)   89
6.2   Complex public health interventions   90
6.3   Formative and process evaluation for CPE   92
6.4   Evaluation designs for complex programs   95
6.5   Challenges in conducting CPEs   97
6.6   Summary   102
References   102

CHAPTER 7

Evaluation methods for program replication,
dissemination and institutionalisation   104

7.1   Stages in assessing the significance of programs   105
7.2   Replication (intervention demonstration)   107
7.3   Dissemination   111
7.4   Institutionalisation   114
7.5   Summary   116
      References   117

CHAPTER 8

Evidence, practice, policy and the critical practitioner   119

8.1   Getting evidence into practice   119
8.2   Getting evidence into policy   123
8.3   Critical appraisal of research and evaluation evidence   124
8.4   Concluding comments: evaluation—art and science   128
      References   129

Appendices   130
Glossary   141
Index   149

list of tables and figures

TABLES

Chapter 1

Table 1.1   Hypothetical logic model: planning a health promotion program to improve healthy food in school canteens   15

Chapter 2

Table 2.1   The differences and similarities between practitioner and scientific perspectives of health promotion programs   21

Table 2.2   Case studies of research illustrating the stages in the model using different health promotion interventions   30

Chapter 3

Table 3.1   Examples of the uses of formative evaluation in health promotion   43

Chapter 4

Table 4.1   Practical tasks in carrying out process evaluation tasks   55
Table 4.2   Examples of process evaluation (PE)   57

Chapter 5

Table 5.1   Examples of research design   72
Table 5.2   Sampling methods used in the evaluation of health promotion interventions   76
Table 5.3   Measurement at different stages of program evaluation   85

Chapter 6

Table 6.1   Published examples of CPEs showing 'complexity' in
formative, process and impact evaluation   100

Chapter 7

Table 7.1   Replication and dissemination examples   110

Chapter 8

Table 8.1   Examples of systematic reviews of health
promotion evidence   126

Appendices

Table A2.1   Examples of statistical techniques and analysis in a
hypothetical (and effective) weight-loss intervention   131

Table A3.1   Some examples of techniques and methods used to
assess measurement reliability and validity   133

FIGURES

Chapter 1

Figure 1.1   The planning and evaluation cycle   2
Figure 1.2   Health promotion actions and outcomes   8
Figure 1.3   Theoretical distribution over time of outcomes
from health promotion interventions   12

Chapter 2

Figure 2.1   Building evidence for public health programs:
stages of research and evaluation   24

Chapter 3

Figure 3.1   Stages showing formative, process and impact/
outcome evaluations   39

Chapter 4

Figure 4.1   Advanced statistical modelling in process evaluation:
            understanding how interventions work through
            mediator and moderator analyses   60

Chapter 5

Figure 5.1   The evaluation process   66
Figure 5.2   Quantitative evaluation designs for individual
            programs (stage 3 of Figure 2.1), ranked from
            'most scientific' experimental designs to less scientific
            'pre-experimental' designs   74
Figure 5.3   Reliability (reproducibility) and responsiveness of
            measurement   83

Chapter 6

Figure 6.1   Complex interventions: planning and
            evaluation stages   92

Chapter 7

Figure 7.1   Stages in scaling up interventions to achieve
            population health   106
Figure 7.2   Conceptual framework for research replication and
            dissemination   107

Chapter 8

Figure 8.1   Variation in the use of evidence in health promotion:
            planned, responsive and reactive practice   120

about the authors

Adrian Bauman is Sesquicentenary Professor of Public Health and Health Promotion at the University of Sydney, Australia. He directs the WHO Collaborating Centre on Physical Activity, Nutrition and Obesity, which has a major interest in chronic disease prevention. He has taught health promotion research methods and program evaluation to public health students for 30 years, and has applied these principles in his population health research program. His recent research interests are in research translation and in evaluating scaled-up health promotion interventions at the population level.

Don Nutbeam is Vice-Chancellor of the University of Southampton, UK, and a Professor of Public Health. He was formerly Head of Public Health in the UK Department of Health.

Acknowledgments

Several people have contributed to the development of *Evaluation in a Nutshell*. We would like to acknowledge the contribution of Bill Bellew and Lesley King for their constructive comments and advice on early drafts of this edition of the book.

preface

This book is for students of health promotion and for health promotion practitioners. *Evaluation in a Nutshell* is intended to equip the reader with the ability to understand, interpret and assess the quality of published research, and to excite interest in evaluation and promote further study that will lead to the development of core skills in evaluation. It provides foundation knowledge and recommended further reading.

In writing this book, we have drawn on many years of experience in conducting evaluations of health promotion programs, working with health promotion practitioners and teaching public health students. From this experience we recognise the need for students and practitioners to understand the basic principles of evaluation and the application of these principles in evaluation design, whether for the purpose of conducting an evaluation or for assessing the work of others.

Any review of published research will reveal that not all health promotion programs are equally successful in achieving their goals and objectives. Experience tells us that programs are most likely to be successful when the determinants of a health problem are well understood; when the needs and motivations of the target population are addressed; and when the context in which the program is being implemented is taken into account. That is, the intervention 'fits' the problem.

Similarly, in developing an evaluation design for a health promotion program, the evaluation design needs to fit the circumstances of the program. Programs can be evaluated in a range of ways, may demand differing levels of resources and may use various evaluation designs. This book illustrates how evaluation questions change as a program evolves, and shows how programs that are truly innovative need close scrutiny and highly structured and comprehensive evaluation. On the other hand, programs that have previously been shown to work in a variety of circumstances, and are low-cost and low-risk, will require more modest monitoring for the purposes of accountability and quality control. The evaluation of projects with tightly defined objectives in a controlled environment will be different to that of multi-component, long-term programs.

Evaluations must be tailored to suit the activity and circumstances of individual programs: no single method or design will be 'right' for all programs.

Evaluation in a Nutshell introduces the strategic and technical issues in evaluation and discusses some of the practical and scientific challenges related to the evaluation of health promotion programs. The book takes a real-life public health perspective. Even for experienced researchers and practitioners, the book provides a useful prompt on key issues, as well as guidance on how to organise and conduct evaluation studies.

introduction

Evaluation is the formal process of judging the 'value' of something. In health promotion, an evaluation will determine the extent to which a program has achieved its desired health outcomes and will assess the contribution of the different processes that were applied to achieve these outcomes. Scientists, health practitioners, politicians and the wider community all have different views on what represents 'value' from a health promotion program, how success should be defined and what should be measured. For example:

- Policy-makers and budget managers need to judge the likely success of programs in order to make decisions about how to allocate resources and to be accountable for these decisions. Success is often defined by the relationship between financial investment and the achievement of health outcomes in the short term.

- Health practitioners need to judge the likely and actual success of a program in achieving its defined health outcomes in 'real-life' situations, so that they know that their work is effective and understand what needs to be done to ensure successful implementation. Success may be defined in terms of the effectiveness of the program in achieving health outcomes, the practicality of implementation, program sustainability and the maintenance of health gains in the longer term.

- The community that is to benefit from health promotion action may place great value on the processes through which a program is conducted, particularly on whether the program is participatory and addresses priorities that the community itself has identified. Success may be defined in terms of relevance to perceived needs and providing opportunities for community participation.

- Academic researchers need to judge a program's success (or failure) in order to contribute to the science of health promotion and improve health promotion practice. Success may be defined in terms of the effects identified through rigorous study designs and measured through quantifiable and validated outcomes, and where the expected effects are theoretically based.

These perspectives are distinct but not mutually exclusive. In each perspective, success is judged through improved health outcomes, yet each differs greatly in the emphasis given to the cost, practicality and processes involved in achieving these outcomes. Correspondingly, there is a vast spectrum of approaches used to evaluate health promotion programs. These range from highly structured, methodology-driven evaluations that focus strongly on the measurement of outcomes through to much less rigid, highly participatory forms of evaluation.

As practitioners, we need to be accountable for what we do and we need to make explicit what we expect to achieve through the investments that are made in health promotion interventions. All programs can benefit from some form of evaluation, but not all require the same intensity of evaluation nor use the same criteria for success. Innovative programs using a costly or controversial intervention for the first time need close scrutiny with comprehensive evaluation. Programs that have been proven to work, and are low-cost and uncontroversial, require monitoring for the purposes of accountability.

This book aims to:

■ provide an overview and a simple classification system for the evaluation of a health promotion program;

■ distinguish between formative, process, impact and outcome evaluation;

■ consider the relative strengths of qualitative and quantitative research methods;

■ provide practical guidance on when and how to evaluate programs, and the range of evaluation designs and research methods that can be used to evaluate different project and program types;

■ consider how best to 'measure' health promotion activity and outcomes;

■ provide a practical glossary of terms used in health promotion program evaluation;

■ refer the reader to sources of further information.

Updates to the examples and tables in this book will be made available at www.mhhe.com/au/bauman2e.

1

Planning for evaluation

This chapter introduces the purposes and functions of evaluation and describes the stages in planning and implementing a health promotion program or intervention. These range from defining the problem and developing solutions to planning and implementing programs. Each stage is linked to the evaluation methods described in this book.

Evaluation should be included during the planning stage as an integral part of the development of a **project** or program. It is far more difficult to 'add' the evaluation in at later stages, after the critical decisions on program design and execution have been made.

Successful evaluation of a program is more likely if:

- a thorough analysis of a health problem and its distribution in a population is conducted (this will indicate the scope for intervention);
- there are clearly defined, logical and feasible program **goals** and **objectives** related to the initial analysis;
- formative assessment is used to develop an **intervention**, giving sufficient attention to the materials, resources and human capacity required for successful implementation;
- the intervention is implemented as planned;
- the project or program is of sufficient size, duration and sophistication to be proven effective or ineffective in relation to its goals and objectives;
- there is clear direction on how the evaluation is to be conducted and what is to be measured;
- the evaluation provides sufficient relevant information to those deciding the program's value.

Achieving these conditions for successful evaluation is challenging, but more likely if a structured approach to planning is adopted.

Planning models are commonly used in the development and management of contemporary health promotion. Such models support evidence-led practice and provide a foundation for systematic evaluation by specialist evaluators, when this is feasible and funded. Some models of planning use population, and individual enablers, facilitators and barriers, to identify the best approach to project planning (Green & Kreuter 2005); others use planning models to specify the intervention components to be delivered.

Using a model enables those planning a project or program to structure the various sources of information that have guided the development of the intervention, and to consider in a logical sequence the likelihood of achieving the program goals and objectives through each step and strategy planned for the program. A model provides a structured description of how the impacts of, and outcomes from, a health promotion intervention develop over time and also provides a sound foundation for the evaluation of an intervention (see Chapter 5).

Figure 1.1 presents the health promotion planning and evaluation 'cycle' used in the companion volume to this book, *Theory in a Nutshell: A Practical Guide to Health Promotion Theories* (Nutbeam et al. 2010). This describes the various stages in the planning, implementation and evaluation of a health

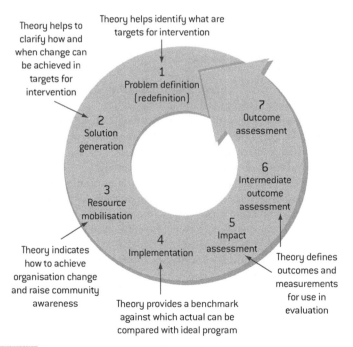

Figure 1.1 The planning and evaluation cycle

promotion program, in the form of a cycle. In this chapter, we consider each of these stages in turn.

1.1   Problem definition: starting at the end

A wide range of information can be used to define a health problem and generate potentially effective solutions. This may include routinely collected epidemiological, demographic and behavioural and social information, but may be enhanced by focused local community needs assessments. At this *information-gathering* stage, it is important to consider:

- what is the overall magnitude of the problem—how many people in the target population are likely to have the problem or be affected by it?
- how prevalent is the problem in various subgroups (for example, older adults, adolescents and people from socially disadvantaged or culturally diverse populations)?
- what is the public health impact of the problem—how serious are the consequences of the problem for the individuals affected and the population as a whole (for example, does it contribute to disability, reduced quality of life or reduced mental health, and does it increase health service usage and costs or contribute to premature death)?
- does it have any impact outside health (on the environment, economic effects or effects on other sectors)?
- what is the potential for intervention—can some factors or conditions be changed that will have an impact on the problem (these may be behavioural, social or environmental, or relate to improved health services)?
- what evidence is there that, if there is potential to intervene to change risks or conditions, this may produce the desired improvements in public health?
- what evidence is there that the community recognises the problem and gives priority to addressing it?

1.2   Planning a solution

The second stage in the cycle prompts analysis of potential solutions, leading to the development of a **program plan** and/or individual project component plans that specify the interventions to be employed, as well as the sequence of activity. Planning for a program will inevitably be more complex and multifaceted than planning for a more limited individual project, because it involves clearer sequencing and the use of a wider range of measures for success. The differences between projects and program evaluation are discussed in greater detail in Chapters 3 and 4.

This stage in the planning process indicates how and when change might be achieved in the target variable (population, organisation or policy). The processes of change in the program are identified, leading to the selection of effective interventions to achieve change and to the timing and sequencing of interventions designed to achieve maximum effect. This stage in the planning process can be supported by the use of techniques such as *intervention mapping* (IM) and **logic models**. These techniques describe how the project or program elements are expected to work, involving the structured, systematic description of the intervention and the changes that a project or program is intended to bring about, and defining what will happen during a program, in what order and with what anticipated effects. These planning processes and techniques are also part of **formative evaluation** (the steps required before a program is launched), described in Chapter 3.

A theoretical framework or model often underpins the planning of health promotion programs, guiding the project or program's content. These theories can be considered using a socio-ecological framework and may include strategies to influence a range of people, from individuals and small groups to communities, environments and policies. Further information on theories and models in health promotion practice can be found in Nutbeam, Harris & Wise (2010). A review of health promotion programs shows that a wide range of potential intervention methods can be used. A discrete project based on the use of a single method (such as education) in a well-defined setting (such as a school) may make detailed use of individual behaviour change theory, and the tasks of evaluation will usually be clear. In a more comprehensive program that uses different intervention strategies in different settings and that is directed at different target populations, the task of evaluation is generally more complex and contentious. The interdependence of the various health promotion actions makes it difficult to assess their individual contributions and poses real problems in the choice of evaluation methods and the analysis of results. These challenges in **evaluation design** and the differences in evaluating *projects* and *programs* are considered more fully in Chapters 5 and 6.

Decisions about what represents the best starting point and how to combine the different interventions will be guided by established health promotion theory, evidence from past programs and the experience of others, and knowledge of the local context in which the program will be implemented.

The development of program strategies that incorporate the right combination of actions in the right sequence completes the planning stage of the program and should link clearly and logically to the project or program outcomes that were identified in the first stage of planning. Some modification of the **objectives** may be required at this stage, together with refinements to the measures used to evaluate the short-term impact of a program. The measurement of impact and outcome is addressed in more detail in Chapter 5.

It is essential to define clearly the planned optimal structure and sequencing of the intervention in the second step of the planning process. This definition provides a point of reference for evaluating the process of implementation that has led to progress (or lack of progress) in achieving program goals and objectives. This is described in more detail in Chapter 3 and is a compulsory element of any program evaluation. This process provides key information that will be very useful to practitioners in refining and reproducing future interventions.

1.3   Creating the right conditions for the successful implementation of programs

This stage (stage 3 in Figure 1.1) is not only concerned with obtaining the resources (such as money, staff and materials) required for the successful implementation of a project or program. It is also concerned with the need to build capacity in a community or organisation to enable an intervention to be introduced and sustained, and to generate and maintain the community and political support necessary for successful implementation. It will usually involve different types of formative evaluation, testing and piloting of interventions to be used as a part of the program. Formative evaluation is described in more detail in Chapter 3.

In some circumstances, either the resource assessment or formative evaluation of methods and materials may show that the available resources or community response do not match what is needed. It will then be necessary to reformulate the program objectives to better fit available resources and/or to clarify the types of action required to secure the level of community and political support necessary to generate essential resources and opportunities for action. This planning stage is important whether the intervention is a simple, time-limited project or a more complex, long-term program with multiple components.

Insufficient attention to this phase in the development of a program, including the pre-testing of methods and materials, is a common reason for program failure. This is especially true when program delivery may involve working through partners, such as schools, work sites and different government agencies.

1.4   Planning for the implementation of health promotion projects and programs

The next stage is planning for implementation (stage 4 in Figure 1.1). At this planning stage, the primary aim is to ensure that a program is likely to be implemented as closely as possible to the original plan, recognising that implementation in 'real-life' conditions will often require adaptation. Good record-keeping to assess the process of implementation is the key evaluation task at this stage. This will enable subsequent examination of program **fidelity** (the extent to which a program was implemented as planned) and the relationship between program implementation and subsequent observed outcomes. Further information on **process evaluation** is described in Chapter 4.

There may be pressure to implement projects with insufficient resources, within time frames that are too short or in communities that are not ready for the intervention. Such projects may happen, but such pressure often leads to incomplete project implementation and tends to produce incomplete evidence on the program's **effectiveness**.

As we have seen, the implementation of a project or program may involve one or multiple strategies or components to achieve the program objectives and goals that were identified through the initial analysis of the problem and its **determinants**. Traditionally, health promotion interventions have relied heavily on methods designed to promote individual behaviour change through public education or mass communication aimed at improving knowledge and changing attitudes. Increasingly, however, health promotion programs involve other forms of intervention designed to influence the social, environmental and economic factors that determine health. This requires working through professional groups and directly with communities in different ways to mobilise social action, as well as advocating for political and organisational change. Combining the delivery of different interventions and securing the necessary partnerships to achieve desired **health promotion outcomes** are among the major challenges for practitioners.

1.5   Health promotion actions and outcomes

It is important to identify and define a range of measurable *outcomes* that form the basis for a program plan. These outcomes range from the direct 'impact' of health promotion interventions in the short term to **health outcomes** in the longer term. These levels of program effects are shown in Figure 1.1 as stages 5–7. They provide an overview of the relationship between the 'processes' of health promotion and the different types of impact and outcome that such interventions might produce.

A comprehensive health promotion program (see Chapter 6) might consist of multiple interventions targeted at achieving different types of outcome in the shorter and longer term. A shorter term health promotion project might focus on achieving a smaller subset of health promotion outcomes. Figure 1.2 shows a typology that characterises these different health promotion actions and the subsequent measures that can be used to assess their impact and outcomes.

Working from the end-points on the right-hand side of the model in Figure 1.2, *health and social outcomes* reflect the end-points of health and preventive interventions. Thus, outcomes such as quality of life, functional independence and equity have the highest value in the model. Some health outcomes are also more narrowly defined in terms of disease and physical and mental health status. For example, for an HIV-prevention program the primary health outcome would be to reduce HIV infection and AIDS-related mortality rates.

Intermediate health outcomes represent the *determinants* (immediate antecedents) of health and social outcomes. These include personal behaviours that provide protection from disease or injury (such as physical activity) or increase risk of ill health (such as tobacco use) and are represented as *healthy lifestyles* in the model. The physical environment can limit people's access to facilities or represent a direct hazard to their physical safety, and economic and social conditions can enhance or limit people's ability to adopt recommended behaviours. These determinants are represented as *healthy environments*. Access to, and appropriate use of, preventive services are acknowledged as an important determinant of health status and are represented as *effective preventive health services*.

Thus, for example, a multi-component program designed to reduce HIV infection rates in the long term might have a *project* component targeted at a sex worker population. In this case, the project might be directed towards:

- achieving preventive behaviours (safe sex) among the target population;
- delivering services that provide access to HIV testing and affordable HIV treatment for the target population.

Health promotion actions	Health promotion outcomes [outcomes of the process of intervention]	Intermediate health outcomes [program impact, or short-term outcomes]	Social health outcomes [long-term outcomes]
Education Examples include patient education, school education and broadcast media communication	*Health literacy* Measures include health-related knowledge, attitude, motivation, behavioural intentions, personal skills and self-efficacy	*Healthy lifestyles* Measures include tobacco use, physical activity, food choices and alcohol and illicit drug use	*Social outcomes* Measures include quality of life, functional independence, social capital and equity
Social mobilisation Examples include community development, group facilitation and technical advice	*Social action and influence* Measures include community participation, community empowerment, social norms and public opinion	*Effective preventive health services* Measures include access to and provision of relevant and preventive services	
Advocacy Examples include lobbying, political organisation and activism, and overcoming bureaucratic inertia	*Healthy public policy and organisational practices* Measures include policy statements, legislation, regulation and resource allocation organisational practices	*Healthy environments* Measures include safe physical environment, supportive economic and social conditions, good food supply and restricted access to tobacco/alcohol	*Health outcomes* Measures include reduced morbidity, reduced disability and avoidable mortality

Figure 1.2 Health promotion actions and outcomes

At the previous stage, *health promotion outcomes* (shown in Figure 1.2) refer to modifiable personal, social and environmental factors that lead to the determinants of health (intermediate health outcomes). These may represent the immediate results of planned health promotion activities. Thus, they include measures of the cognitive and social skills that determine the ability of individuals to gain access to, understand and use health information (**health literacy** in the model). Examples of health promotion outcomes would include improved health knowledge and an understanding of where to go and what to do to gain access to health services and other support. *Social action and influence* includes organised efforts to promote or enhance the actions and control of social groups over the determinants of health. This includes the mobilisation of human and material resources in social action to overcome structural barriers to health, enhance social support and reinforce social norms conducive to health. Examples of outcomes range from improved social 'connectedness' and social support to improved community empowerment.

Healthy environments are largely determined by *healthy public policy and organisational practices*. Policy-determined legislation, funding, regulations and incentives significantly influence organisational practices. Thus, examples of health promotion outcomes here might be changes to health and social policies that lead to improvements in services, social benefits, the built environment and housing. These would influence organisational practices and redirect resource allocation to support environments conducive to health.

Using the HIV-prevention project as an example, health promotion outcomes could include:

■ improving health literacy by raising levels of accurate knowledge about HIV prevention and improving skills and confidence to put into practice recommended behaviours in challenging circumstances among the target population;

■ facilitating a more supportive environment through social action, to improve commitment to safe sex practices in commercial sex establishments, and to support access to condoms and other preventive behaviours;

■ improving health policy and services by providing more facilities for, and better access to, HIV testing and regular health checks among the target population.

Figure 1.2 also indicates three health promotion actions—what to do, as distinct from what outcomes are achieved. *Education* consists primarily of the creation of opportunities for learning that are intended to raise levels of personal health literacy and thereby increase the capacity of individuals and communities to act to improve and protect their health. *Social mobilisation* is action taken in partnership with individuals or social groups to mobilise social and material resources for health. **Advocacy** is action taken on behalf of individuals and/or communities to overcome structural barriers to the achievement of health.

In the example of HIV prevention, these health promotion actions would include, for example, the direct education of sex workers; advocacy on their behalf with operators of commercial sex establishments; and training of health professionals to advocate for and provide HIV testing and treatment services.

Another example of this hierarchy of actions and outcomes can be considered for smoking-prevention programs among teenagers. Social and health outcomes include reduced tobacco-related morbidity and mortality, but these outcomes may come decades after the original health promotion program. Intermediate outcomes include reduced smoking rates and higher quit rates among adolescents. Health promotion outcomes would include measures of intention to not smoke, changes to social and peer norms around smoking, and policies restricting cigarette advertising or restricting purchases (as in proof of age requirements). In the far left-hand column of Figure 1.2, *health promotion actions* in this example would comprise the *education* of young people concerning the negative consequences of smoking; the **social mobilisation** of parents and other social role models to make smoking less socially attractive and acceptable to young people; and *advocacy* for legislative action to reduce access to tobacco and exposure to tobacco advertising.

Figure 1.2 can be used to illustrate not only the linkages *between* the different levels of outcomes but also those *within* levels. For example, among the intermediate outcomes, *action to create healthy environments* may be a direct determinant of social and health outcomes (for example, by producing a safe working and living environment or improving equity in access to resources), and also separately influence healthy lifestyles, for example, by improving access to healthy food or restricting access to tobacco products. There is a dynamic relationship between these different outcomes and the three health promotion actions; it is not the static, linear relationship that the model in Figure 1.2 might suggest.

By starting in this way, the beginning of the planning process is firmly focused on the end-point outcomes and the shorter term measures that are logically related to their achievement. Starting planning with the end-points prompts a thorough and logical analysis of the linkages between intervention and outcome. This phase ensures that there is a clear definition of who or what is the target of the intervention (sub-population group, environmental or organisational element) and what outcomes will be sought. The early definition of these outcomes and consideration of how they might be measured form the important first stage of the evaluation process. The principles of measurements, and selection methods, are described further in Chapter 5.

1.6   Evaluation

Different types of evaluation tasks occur at each stage of the cycle shown in Figure 1.1. These start with *formative evaluation*, a set of activities designed to develop and pre-test program materials and methods (see Chapter 3); and *process evaluation*, a set of activities directed towards assessing progress in program implementation (see Chapter 4).

Health promotion interventions have different types of *impact* and different *outcomes* over time. Change in the different types of outcome will occur according to different timescales, depending on the nature of the intervention and the type of social or health problem being addressed. As a consequence, different evaluation methods are used to measure impact and outcome at different stages in the life of a program.

Impact evaluation measures the short-term effects that are predicted and defined during the planning stage of the program. These impact measures are termed *health promotion outcomes* in Figure 1.2. These health promotion outcomes are intended to lead to subsequent change in *intermediate health outcomes*, for example, in behaviours and environments, in ways that will ultimately improve health and social outcomes in the model. Outcome assessment involves the measurement of individual behaviour or changes to the social, economic and environmental conditions that determine health. Figure 1.2 provides examples of these intermediate outcomes. The assessment of *social and health outcomes* is the end-point assessment of health promotion.

Figure 1.3 illustrates how a comprehensive set of health promotion interventions might produce different outcomes over time. This model was originally developed to illustrate likely progress over a five-year period in a comprehensive, community-based heart disease–prevention program. Thus the 'units of time' are years and the model shows how, after one year, the program impact could be measured mainly in terms of increased community awareness and participation in intervention components. By the third year, good progress in achieving short-term program impacts (health promotion outcomes) should be measurable, alongside peak-level community awareness and participation. Early progress in achieving intermediate outcomes (such as behavioural risks) should also be measurable. After five years, major progress in these intermediate outcomes should be observable and early impact

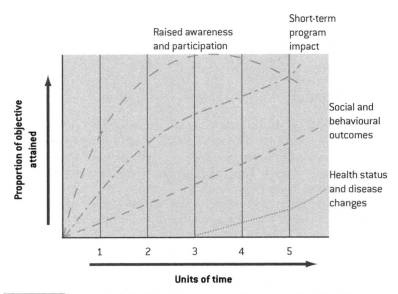

Figure 1.3 Theoretical distribution over time of outcomes from health promotion interventions

on disease outcomes may also be observable. This model can be useful in explaining the timescales required to achieve different levels of impact and outcome to funders and decision-makers. This can be invaluable in managing expectations and promoting fairness in accountability for success over time.

The model in Figure 1.3 can be adapted to fit different types and intensities of intervention. For example, an intensive public education project to promote uptake of a new childhood vaccine may achieve very rapid progress in raising awareness, achieving behaviour change (a simple, one-off action is required) and health outcomes (reduced rates of vaccine-preventable disease in the population), all within a matter of months. Similarly, a successful smoking-cessation intervention for pregnant women or a falls-prevention trial among the elderly could rapidly demonstrate health outcomes in terms of improved infant birth weight or reduced injuries in older people, respectively. In these examples, the 'units of time' may be months, not years.

Practitioners and evaluators are still challenged by unreasonable expectations from impatient policy-makers and funders. Explaining the complexity of interventions and the time lag between intervention and observable effects can often prove challenging for health promotion practitioners and evaluators.

1.7 Summary

The planning and evaluation cycle (Figure 1.1) illustrates the different stages and their relationships in the development of a plan of action, implementation of the plan and evaluation of the achievement of desired health outcomes. These processes in turn lead to a re-definition of the priority problems and solutions and hence to a concept of a 'cycle' of planning and evaluation. Because there are several stages, and often a long time delay between implementation and outcome, it is often difficult to demonstrate a causal relationship between health promotion actions and long-term outcomes. So, it is essential that relevant and appropriate measures are used to chart progress at each stage in the process. A systematic approach to planning and using tools such as *logic models* or *intervention maps* (IM) help to unravel some of these complexities, make the identification of relevant indicators of progress more straightforward and support effective communication and expectation management. The use of logic models in program planning is described in Box 1.1.

The cycle summarised in Figure 1.1 will not address all the issues likely to arise in the planning and evaluation of a health promotion program; real-life decision-making never follows such a smooth path. This model is intended as a guide, to be adapted to prevailing circumstances rather than adopted wholesale without critical examination of its usefulness. In reality, few programs have the resources to apply this model in the systematic way described here. For these reasons, it is to identify what is possible, make explicit the program's likely impact and outcomes, and indicate alternative ways to strengthen the intervention. The outcomes illustrated in Figure 1.3 can help in communicating with key stakeholders about reasonable expectations for achievement over time, and can form a basis for periodic program review and accountability.

The explicit communication of these limitations also helps to set realistic public and political expectations, thereby increasing the program's chances of success.

In order to plan and perform a high-quality evaluation, it is important to acknowledge the limitations of what the program can achieve in a range of circumstances.

Box 1.1 Logic models: a method of summarising a program plan

A *logic model* is a summary description of program inputs (human, financial and material resources), the context of the program (those factors that will influence the implementation and impact of the intervention, including the physical environment, social norms and political and community support) and the activities that together make up the intervention (program events, groups, training, social marketing and so on).

A logic model describes how the intervention elements might cause the program to influence health promotion outcomes as well as intermediate and end-point outcomes. In the planning process, a logic model has to be considered a 'live' statement, capable of modification over time in response to changed circumstances and available resources. The development of a logic model can be seen as a final part of the planning phase of a project or program, describing the project or program's conceptual framework and anticipated effects. If any stage is seen as unachievable or unrealistic, then adjustments to the model can occur before that set of activities is implemented.

Intervention mapping (IM) is a similar technique to the logic model, and combines planning with (behavioural) theory and formative evaluation. In essence, there are six stages in IM, starting with needs assessments, qualitative **consultation** and community participation in planning (known as **participatory planning**). IM then defines program goals (as do logic models) and develops structured program and implementation plans. The theoretical framework underpinning the anticipated changes should be identified.

An example of a logic model for health promotion is shown in Table 1.1. The logic model shown describes a hypothetical program with the goal of improving the quality of food sold in school canteens in a region or school district. This example uses health promotion approaches: education and communication, and advocacy for structural reorganisation and policy development. Ideally, each of these health promotion approaches would be tested through formative evaluation with the target populations.

The stages in the logic model in Table 1.1 describe the program inputs, health promotion actions, health promotion outcomes, intermediate health outcomes (impact evaluation), and health and social outcomes. The planning process defines the anticipated changes for each level in the logic model. For example, the creation of curricula and development of resources are indicators of success in health promotion actions; the implementation of education programs and distribution of resources are health promotion outcomes; and changes in behaviour by students are among the proposed indicators of the impact of the program. Mapping these levels of proposed change as part of the pre-intervention planning provides a detailed set of evaluation indicators to be developed.

Table 1.1 Hypothetical logic model: planning a health promotion program to improve healthy food in school canteens

Resources and inputs	Delivery of intervention: state education department/school councils or boards; local public health department [health promotion practitioners]; school parent and teacher groups			
Activities	Education	Communication	Organisational development	Intersectoral/policy development
Inputs	Teacher time; parents; canteen managers and suppliers.	Teachers, parent and teacher committees, marketing professionals; media chosen [e.g. billboards].	Planning meetings; formation of a steering group; garnering resources.	Within-school re-orientation to health and nutrition as priority issues; reach out to parents; food suppliers.
Activities [health promotion actions]	Writing of best-practice curriculum for 'healthy eating' among teenagers.	Development of media resources [formative evaluation testing with students]; campaign materials and posters for school canteens.	Planning meetings held; partnership developed; planning/logic model developed.	School council/board makes policy changes regarding healthy nutrition offered in canteens.
Outputs [health promotion outcomes]	Education programs implemented; staff and students aware of program.	Posters in all canteens; teachers aware of and accept program.	Healthy choices approved for canteens; budget and financial model approved.	Steering group works towards implementing policy for healthy canteen choices in schools.
Intermediate health outcomes [impact evaluation]	Attempts at behaviour change; healthy eating choices increased among students.	Parents and teachers have more favourable views of program; parents' advocacy for program increases.	Working groups influence local food environment in schools.	Policies around healthy food choices adopted in schools.
Health and social outcomes	Reduced obesity and cardiovascular risk among children.	Increased sense of school community generalises to other school issues.	Health promotion and education work together around other issues.	Sustained healthy food choices due to widespread policy adoption.

References

Green LW & Kreuter MW 2005, *Health Program Planning: An Educational and Ecological Approach*, 4th edn, McGraw-Hill, New York, NY.

Nutbeam D, Harris E & Wise M 2010, *Theory in a Nutshell: A Practical Guide to Health Promotion Theories*, 3rd edn, McGraw-Hill, Sydney.

Further reading

Glasgow RE, Vogt TM & Boles SM 1999, 'Evaluating the public health impact of health promotion interventions: the RE-AIM framework', *American Journal of Public Health*, vol. 89, no. 9, pp. 1322–7.

Nutbeam D 1998, 'Evaluating health promotion: progress, problems and solutions', *Health Promotion International*, vol. 13, no. 1, pp. 27–44.

Van Koperen TM, Jebb SA, Summerbell CD et al. 2013, 'Characterizing the EPODE logic model: unravelling the past and informing the future', *Obesity Reviews*, vol. 14, no. 2, pp. 162–70.

2

Research and evaluation in health promotion: key stages, methods and types

This chapter provides an overview of the different research methods that support the planning process described in Chapter 1. In particular, the chapter describes differences between research- and practice-based evaluation and explains the use of both quantitative and qualitative methods in evaluation. It summarises the six key stages of evaluation required to build an evidence base for health promotion and public health programs. The chapter summarises the different approaches, which are described in greater detail in later chapters.

Evaluation is not a single action but a set of continuous tasks that starts in the planning phase and continues throughout the implementation and translation of an **intervention** or program. This chapter describes these stages of evaluation and provides an introduction to the types of evaluation required to assess and understand the value and effects of health promotion and public health programs.

2.1   Evaluation methods and types

Health promotion projects and programs range in scope, scale, target population and settings. Four hypothetical examples are described below. These illustrate the differences in scope, size of the target population and differences in the evaluation tasks required:

1. A small project encouraging people attending a regional diabetes clinic to take control of their condition and build skills that enable improved self-management, a feeling of greater control over the disease and its effects and adopting healthier lifestyles.

2. A project encouraging pap smear attendance (a behaviour that reduces the risk of cervical cancer) among a group of women from a particular cultural background living in a defined area.

3. A program promoting healthy eating in a community in a defined region, including mass media education, nutrition education in the school classroom, and a project to introduce healthy menu choices in restaurants, schools and worksites across the target region.

4. A multiple-agency partnership program, including departments of health, urban planning and transport, aiming to use new urban designs for housing and recreational facilities to improve the physical and social environment, enabling and supporting increased physical activity in the community.

There is a distinction between the first two *projects*, which are quite discrete, and the more complex and comprehensive *programs* intended to promote healthy eating and to create supportive conditions for physical activity. The evaluation methods and the measures of outcome required for these four examples will all be different. In the two projects, the target population is well-defined and the intervention is quite self-contained. The evaluation methods most suited to these projects will be described in greater detail in Chapter 5. In the two *programs*, there are multiple forms of intervention, different target populations and considerable dependence on partnership with and between agencies and sectors. The evaluation methods required for these programs are discussed in Chapter 6, as complex program evaluations (CPEs).

It is immediately obvious in these four examples that there is no single, correct approach to evaluation for different forms of intervention. Evaluation of the four examples will differ in terms of the budgets required, length of time available for evaluation, and evaluation designs and research methods used. Customised approaches should be used to plan, implement and evaluate each project or program.

The first example is a project set in a health facility and will involve a small (selected) number of attending individuals receiving a high level of support to develop the skills necessary to manage their condition. A key evaluation challenge here will be measurement, assessing whether or not the skills and self-management practices (for example, self-efficacy and successful self-management) change in those that attend. This may best be assessed by comparing change in these key measures in the intervention population with a group who do not receive the intervention (a control group). Such a project may be amenable to the rigorous scientific research design, allowing for a full assessment of the project's **efficacy**—that is, the extent to which a health promotion intervention is successful under controlled or 'best possible' conditions.

The second example is a project in a multicultural community-based setting, and its success and sustainability will depend on the involvement of the target population in the activity. Evaluation needs to include assessment of the process of engagement with community stakeholders in the cultural group concerned. The evaluation will need to test how well the health promotion workers engage with the community, and how well they develop and deliver the pap smear service for this community. The outcome to be measured is a sustained increase in uptake of pap smears in a targeted group. Such a project may be less amenable to rigorous assessment of *efficacy*, but more likely to provide evidence of *effectiveness*—that is, the extent to which a health promotion intervention is successful in 'real-life' conditions in achieving the impact and outcomes that were predicted in the planning phase of the intervention.

The third example is a program that will include engagement with many different stakeholders in schools, work sites and restaurants; considerable negotiation will be required to define program goals and objectives, and assess how well an optimal program, given available resources, can be delivered to the participating organisations. The outcome to be measured will be the increased availability of healthy food choices in canteens, vending machines and restaurants, and changes in the food choices made by those using the facilities. Assessing the impact of the mass media component of the program may involve community surveys to assess changes in knowledge of, and attitudes towards, healthy eating. Again, this study is more likely to produce evidence of *effectiveness* than *efficacy*.

The fourth example is a program that will involve multiple partnerships. Evaluating the effective functioning of partnerships will be an important part of this evaluation. Assessing the common needs across agencies and defining common program elements are critical first steps, followed by an assessment of how well the agencies work together towards a common task, in this case, the challenge of building health promoting environments over a number of years. The outcomes to be measured may include coalition-building across agencies, changes to urban policy and the built environment, and assessment of the impact of such changes on participation in physical activity in the local community.

The third and fourth examples demonstrate evaluation of complex public health programs (see Chapter 6), as they are comprised of multiple elements and program strategies.

2.2 Balancing scientific design with practical need

Chapter 1 indicates that the concepts of *relevance, efficacy* and *effectiveness* will vary between research scientists, practitioners, policy-makers and members of communities that may be the target of interventions. Health promotion research scientists value optimal design, such as controlled research designs, which aim to increase the 'academic evidence base' through scientific publication of results. These may have best possible research designs and provide evidence of *efficacy*, showing that a project can work under optimal conditions, with motivated staff delivering the program to a highly engaged study population. This may provide good-quality evidence of the true nature of a program's effects, but the evidence may not be generalisable or transferable to the wider community. For example, a project that produced good results in well-managed, 'optimal' conditions for implementation might not produce the same effects if conducted in a poor neighbourhood, with diverse cultural groups or delivered by health practitioners in everyday 'real-life' conditions.

By contrast, when community stakeholders and practitioners manage an evaluation, its design is often more flexible and adaptive, reflecting the less predictable course of many community interventions and the need to adapt to changing circumstances. This will often produce information that practitioners value and may be adaptable for use in other settings (referred to as 'generalisable'), answering questions about the project's usefulness and relevance to its participants. However, this type of evaluation is less likely to produce convincing evidence that a defined intervention led directly to (or 'caused') specific, observed outcomes. (See glossary; this is an example of likely *external validity* or **generalisability** of an intervention, but less good scientific rigour or *internal validity*.)

Table 2.1 summarises key differences in these two perspectives by considering issues of research methods and desired outcomes. For the purposes of illustration, it provides an exaggerated view of these differences in perspective, and there is no suggestion that those interested in advancing scientific understanding are not interested in health promotion practice, or vice versa.

What will become apparent through an examination of the elements in Table 2.1 is that both science and practice are codependent, and are best served by a 'middle way': an integrated approach that involves an evaluation partnership meeting both researcher and practitioner needs.

Such an approach will focus attention on not only the practicality and relevance of an intervention for a specific population, but also the scientific value of a program, and supports collaboration between researcher and practitioner to this end.

Table 2.1 The differences and similarities between practitioner and scientific perspectives of health promotion programs

Function	Practitioner perspective (informs program implementation)	Scientific perspective (provides scientific levels of evidence)
Control of program, resources	Controlled by managers and/or stakeholders; evaluation carried out for accountability to funding agencies; practice-led evaluation.	Researcher/academic investigator-led evaluation; may be externally funded by peer review scientific grants; research goals of furthering knowledge, scientific publication.
Purpose of evaluation	Identify 'effectiveness' of project or program in real-world conditions; may be used to implement and improve programs, not to 'prove' programs; provides evidence on the need for more or different allocation of resources.	Aim to generate scientific evidence for program effects; generate evidence of 'efficacy'; how well does the project or program work in optimal controlled research conditions.
Research methods	**Quantitative** and **qualitative methods**; mixed methods, including various research methods; **triangulate** results. Apply pragmatic mix of evaluation methods based on needs, available funding. Conclusions may include qualitative judgments of practitioners, community, stakeholders.	Usually quantitative methods; optimal statistical techniques and research methods; emphasis on **statistical significance**; conclusions flow logically from results. Attention to methodological issues such as selection **bias** (who participates), measurement **reliability** and **validity**, control for confounding.
Level of evaluation	Strong emphasis on formative evaluation, especially community consultation, needs assessments. Emphasis on process evaluation—monitoring how well the program activities are implemented and delivered; may adapt and improve program in response to process evaluation findings.	Strong emphasis on impact and outcome evaluation and providing 'proof' or evidence of program effects; attention to the adherence to the research protocol.
Research design	Flexible and pragmatic program design to fit the context and target groups addressed by the program.	Tightly controlled research design, with greater measurable focus, may have single outcomes and shorter time frames to assess outcomes.

(continued)

Table 2.1 *continued*

Function	Practitioner perspective (informs program implementation)	Scientific perspective (provides scientific levels of evidence)
Single focus versus comprehensive approach	Often multi-component programs, with partnerships and interagency collaboration usual. Duration: several years and interventions at multiple levels.	May be single component or single focus for intervention in a specific group; often theory-based or testing a specific theoretical approach; follow-up usually short-term, typically around 6 to 12 months.
Uses of results	Program failure leads to program improvement and modification; program failure may disappoint decision-makers or the community such that funding or support are withdrawn. Successful programs lead to efforts at **dissemination** more widely; to get the program used and adopted in other communities or settings.	Contributes to scientific pool of evidence around the effectiveness of that type of intervention. Successful programs need **replication** in different settings to examine if similar effects are produced. Programs that show repeated success are amenable to [1] **meta-analysis** to summarise results and [2] dissemination trials.

Partnerships between funding agencies, researchers, practitioners, communities, stakeholders or participants improve the breadth of the evidence available from health promotion programs. Health promotion science and practice can only advance if we know how and why programs work, whether they are meeting the needs of communities and stakeholders, and whether they pass scientific scrutiny and critical judgment. Each element is important; concentrating on one to the exclusion of others will make what is found less useful.

2.3   Stages of evaluation

Figure 2.1 on page 24 provides the central framework for this book. It shows the research and evaluation questions that are addressed stage by stage in the planning, evaluation and dissemination of health promotion projects and programs.

The early stages relate to the development and testing of an intervention, and later stages are concerned with the dissemination and adoption of effective or proven individual programs. Stages 1 and 2 indicate the importance of a range of different forms of descriptive research in the development of an intervention plan, as well as *formative evaluation* of the development of program components (see Chapter 3 for more detail).

Stage 3 represents the careful evaluation of a relatively discrete individual project or a more complex program (see Chapter 5). This includes *process evaluation*, and assessment of the impact and outcome of the individual program (**outcome evaluation**). This type of study is intended to provide the best evidence of efficacy (where feasible) or its potential effectiveness in 'real-life' conditions, which will facilitate decisions about whether it warrants further testing and wider dissemination.

At stage 4, the intervention is replicated and tested in other settings to assess, for example, whether or not it works as well in other populations or other places; there is a greater focus on whether it is 'generalisable'. Gradually, the emphasis in the model on assessing the effectiveness of individual program evaluation elements is replaced by a focus on the processes of implementation and the extent to which successful implementation can be reproduced to achieve the same outcomes.

By stage 5, the research emphasis is on the dissemination process and on maximising the population-wide **reach** of the intervention, **scaling up** a program to maximise its potential public health benefit. This requires a focus on understanding the processes of implementation in different settings and a relative decrease in focus on assessing outcomes. Stage 6, when a program is already widely adopted, is the phase of program sustainability and maintenance; this phase highlights the importance of continued monitoring of quality processes, but distinguishes between this more routine quality-assurance process and the more formal research and evaluation methods required in the earlier stages.

The model demonstrates that different, but connected, research methods contribute to health promotion planning and evaluation. These range from epidemiological studies (stage 1) to program planning and formative evaluation to test community responses (stage 2), to formal evaluation trials of programs (stage 3) and studies of the process of program replication and dissemination (stages 4–6). Through this staged process, interventions can be optimally developed and systematically tested and, if found to be effective, widely replicated to maximise their public health benefit.

Although not everyone can be an expert in all of the research methodologies implied in this multi-stage evaluation model, it is important to understand the distinct forms of research that support health promotion, and to be able to critically analyse the quality and relevance of different types of research. Each stage is considered in turn and illustrated using published case studies from the literature (shown in Table 2.2 on pages 30–2).

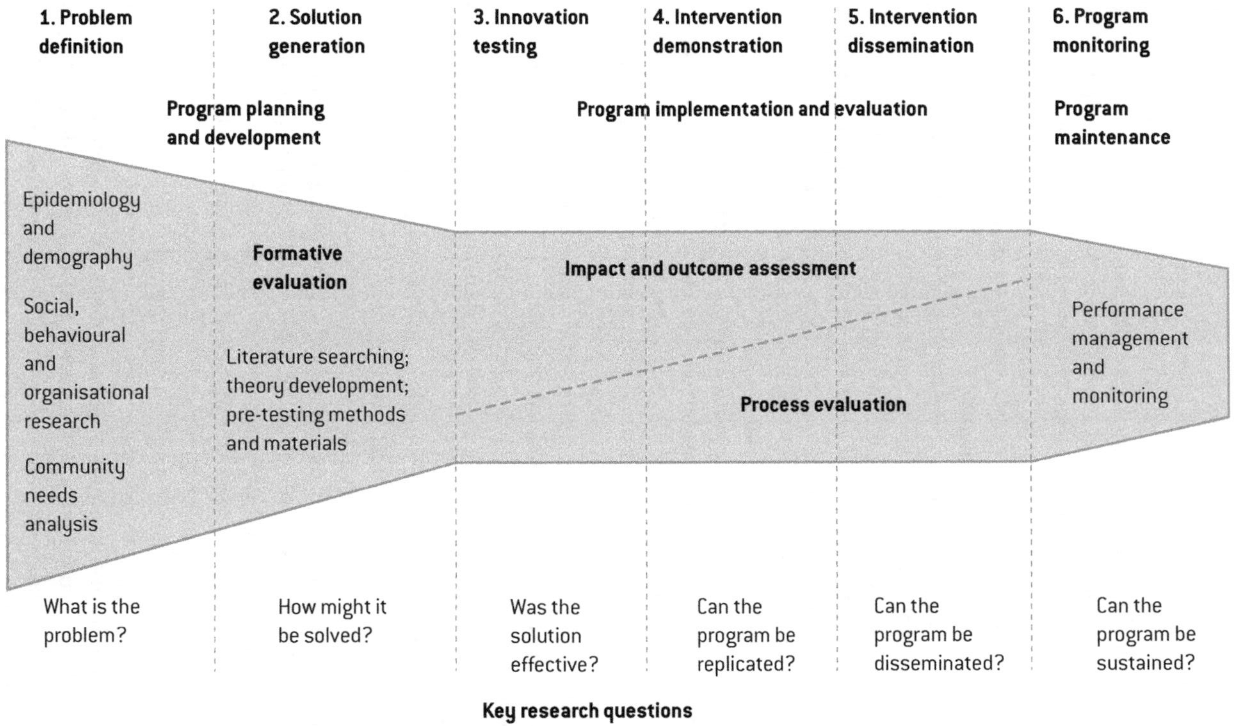

1. Problem definition	2. Solution generation	3. Innovation testing	4. Intervention demonstration	5. Intervention dissemination	6. Program monitoring
Program planning and development		**Program implementation and evaluation**			**Program maintenance**
	Formative evaluation	**Impact and outcome assessment**			
			Process evaluation		**Performance management and monitoring**
Epidemiology and demography	Literature searching; theory development; pre-testing methods and materials				
Social, behavioural and organisational research					
Community needs analysis					
What is the problem?	How might it be solved?	Was the solution effective?	Can the program be replicated?	Can the program be disseminated?	Can the program be sustained?

Key research questions

Figure 2.1 Building evidence for public health programs: stages of research and evaluation

Problem definition (stage 1)

This stage concerns the use of different forms of descriptive data used in program planning. In particular, it requires familiarity with routine epidemiological data (such as causes of mortality and morbidity, and the **prevalence** of identifiable risks to health in populations). Two specialised sub-disciplines, **behavioural epidemiology** (the use of epidemiological methods to understand the origins and determinants of health-related behaviours) and *social epidemiology* (which explores evidence for socioeconomic and structural causes for preventable ill health) may be important at this stage of problem definition, as this research explores the importance (size and severity) of a health issue and investigates the potential causes (determinants) of the problem and the scope for a preventive or health promotion intervention. It may also be useful to conduct community needs assessments at this stage to identify community concerns and priorities; to identify access points to reach key individuals and populations; and to enable more direct community participation in problem definition and solution generation. In combination, information gathered during this stage identifies the major health problems experienced within a defined population, the known causes of these problems and the scope for change in those causal and contributory factors.

For example, Case study 1 in Table 2.2 on page 30 shows an international study of physical inactivity from adult populations in 20 countries. The study identified countries that had lower rates of participation in physical activity and showed how this differed by gender, age and education within a country. This study identified the magnitude of the problem of physical inactivity in all countries, but specifically identified differences between countries that are of relevance to policy-makers working within a country or internationally. The need for physical-activity promotion and strategies could then be prioritised within each country and compared to the prevalence of other non-communicable disease (NCD) risks, such as poor diet and tobacco use.

At this stage in the process, important decisions need to be made concerning the scope of an intervention, to determine whether the project will be self-contained; will focus on a specific risk or health determinant or on a small target group or community; or will take a whole-population approach. In addition, will it comprise a single strategy or consist of a comprehensive, complex program of activities designed to bring about change in the multiple determinants of the health problem?

Solution generation (stage 2)

This stage also draws on social and behavioural research to improve understanding of target populations, and the range of personal, social and environmental and organisational characteristics that may be modifiable to form the basis for intervention. This stage will often involve specific evaluation tasks, including formal qualitative research methods with the target population and/or **pilot testing** intervention of components. These methods of *formative evaluation* are described in Chapter 3. At this stage, the use of theory may help to explain and predict change in individuals, social groups, organisations and the political process. Theories and models are useful in identifying and testing plausible methods for achieving change and assessing the potential for general application in different settings and with different population groups. More information on intervention theory can be found in the partner volume *Theory in a Nutshell: A Practical Guide to Health Promotion Theories* (Nutbeam et al. 2010). This information clarifies the potential content and methods for intervention, and further defines the different needs of populations.

For example, case study 2 in Table 2.2 on page 31 shows a study that examined factors associated with parent views on immunising their pre-school children; the study is an example of the use of 'individual-focused' behaviour change theory, which influences parental decisions. Single and focused behaviours, such as immunisation, especially in health systems where vaccinations are offered free of charge, may be usefully tested using theory. Instead of cross-sectional surveys that only show associations in the data (Bauman 2002), this study examined the factors among parents that predicted whether their children were subsequently vaccinated. The use of 'determinants' rather than cross-sectional **correlates** is better, and the study identified factors that could be usefully emphasised in intervention planning.

Finding a successful, sustainable solution to a defined health problem requires the systematic development and testing of an intervention; these are the necessary outputs of stages 1 and 2 (see Table 2.2 on pages 30–2). This enables program planners to describe the magnitude and importance of a public health problem, identify its social and behavioural determinants and at-risk groups and, following this analysis, propose likely solutions.

Potential solutions can be further developed and tested through *formative evaluation* of initial program components and eventually defined and described as a sequence of activities through the form of a *logic model* or *intervention map* (IM). Evaluation becomes more feasible once such a structured description of a project or program and its anticipated outcomes is in place.

Innovation testing (stage 3)

Ideally, evaluation of a new project or program will go through different stages to establish evidence of its success. Two different, but related, evaluation tasks can be identified: *process evaluation* (assessing the process of implementation) and *impact or outcome evaluation* (assessing the effects of implementation relative to predicted impact and outcomes). These are discussed further below, and also in Chapters 3, 4 and 5. The relative importance of the two evaluation tasks will vary as an intervention goes through different stages of development. Figure 2.1 indicates the logical stages of evaluation beginning with a focused evaluation study to address the question of whether or not an intervention has achieved its desired outcomes: did it work? The function of such a study is to assess the extent to which defined objectives can be achieved, operating in the best possible conditions for success. It is an *efficacy study* if carried out in optimal conditions and an *effectiveness study* if carried out in real-world conditions.

Studies of efficacy and effectiveness need to be developed to meet well-defined methodological standards (see Chapter 5). This type of study tends to fit well with the scientific perspective described in Table 2.1 on pages 21–2. To meet these strict methodological standards, studies that examine the effects of an intervention under optimal conditions are usually quite narrow in focus, and are often developed using a level of resources and methods that are not easily reproduced. This type of study design is generally more achievable for the type of projects described in examples 1 and 2, and much harder to undertake for more complex programs exemplified by examples 3 and 4. Because of the strong focus on evaluation design and the exertion of control over **variables** in the implementation of the intervention, efficacy studies often cannot provide the quality of information about the implementation process that practitioners require to enable them to reproduce the intervention under less than optimal conditions. Hence, there is a need for further study even if an intervention is shown to be successful in the best possible conditions.

Case study 3 in Table 2.2 on page 31 summarises an example of this type of experimental research. This study was an efficacy study testing a community-wide intervention to reduce sexually transmitted infections (STIs) in Peru. Twenty communities were chosen, of which 10 were randomly allocated to be intervention communities. These received a set of interventions targeting STI risk and in particular reaching out to intervene with female sex workers. The study assessed intermediate outcomes, including behaviour change, as well as actual incidence of reported STIs. While the intervention did not reduce the overall incidence of STIs, there were some improvements in subgroups. This study is important in providing new evidence of program effects in a low-to-middle-income country, where rates of STIs and HIV infection may be high and evidence on what to do about them is very limited.

Intervention demonstration (replication) (stage 4)

At the fourth stage, a shift in the relative emphasis given to assessing outcomes and understanding process can be observed. If an intervention achieves the desired outcomes under ideal circumstances, the emphasis of the evaluation changes to consider more closely how to identify the conditions for success. Here the task is to replicate a project in circumstances that are closer to 'real life' and that examine the type of issues that are important to health practitioners, such as the practicality of implementation of a program and the extent to which a program can be adapted to meet variations in local need and circumstances. It represents a shift in focus from demonstrating efficacy under optimal conditions to demonstrating effectiveness in diverse settings, as described earlier.

Replication studies are often relevant to policy-makers, funders and health promotion practitioners, because they indicate that desired outcomes may be achievable in circumstances closer to real life. Specifically, they take account of the contextual variables in health promotion practice and indicate which conditions are essential for the program to be successfully implemented. This type of study, with its balanced emphasis on both process and outcome, often produces more practical guidance about when, where and how an intervention is most likely to be effective. For example, it may indicate the importance of building community engagement, as well as clarifying what resources are required for success. This stage in the evolution of a project or program also offers the opportunity for assessment of costs and benefits more related to real-life conditions—a real test of its *effectiveness*.

Chapter 5 describes the range of issues that should be considered in the design of this type of study, highlighting, for example, the tensions in maintaining the necessary rigour in study design to assess outcomes while ensuring that the intervention is responsive to differences in local circumstances and changes in the operating environment during the life of a project. Because the systems in which we operate are variable, most health promotion interventions also require adaptation to accommodate practical constraints that are encountered during implementation. Evaluation designs and methods must accommodate this need to adapt (Chapter 6).

Case study 4 in Table 2.2 on page 31 provides an example of a replication study. Earlier research trials in the USA and in Norway had demonstrated that curriculum-based interventions using contemporary teaching methods were clearly effective in preventing smoking among adolescents. This study was designed to replicate this type of intervention under usual classroom conditions with 'ordinary' classroom teachers in the UK (Nutbeam et al. 1993). A **cluster randomised controlled trial** was carried out with 4538 students aged 11 and 12 years from 39 schools, to examine whether this intervention worked in real-world conditions. There were a control group and three intervention groups (family smoking prevention; curriculum intervention; both the family and curriculum interventions).

At a two-year follow-up, rates of regular smoking were 11.3 per cent, 14.4 per cent, 12.0 per cent and 10.1 per cent respectively across the four groups, which were not significantly different to each other. The findings from this study were important; replicating previously effective programs in *real-world conditions* may not be as effective as the original trials suggested.

This is an important reminder that we cannot assume that a study that works well in one set of conditions can be transferred to a different environment with equal success.

Intervention dissemination (stage 5)

The fifth stage, dissemination studies, indicates a further shift in emphasis. Here, attention is given to identifying the ways in which successful programs or projects can be widely disseminated. Such studies include those directed at improving understanding of the ways in which communities can be supported to adopt and maintain innovations and build capacity, as well as studies of communities and organisations designed to determine how best to create the necessary conditions for success in different settings.

In these types of study, the balance between outcome and process evaluation has shifted again. The primary focus is on the process of change, and research is directed towards assessing the success of dissemination strategies. This type of information is of great interest not only to practitioners but also to policy-makers and program funders because it helps to define what needs to be done, by whom, to what standard and at what cost. This type of research is least common in the health promotion research literature, partly as a natural consequence of decline in the number of interventions that reach this stage of development (i.e. of proven efficacy and/or effectiveness).

Case study 5 in Table 2.2 on page 32 shows a set of studies around sun protection and skin cancer prevention, targeting outdoor pools in the USA. Initial efficacy trials demonstrated the program could work and subsequent research investigated the dissemination of this intervention to more than 400 pools across the USA (Escoffery et al. 2009, Glanz 2011). The key features of dissemination were explored: what were the facilitators that encouraged program adoption and usage, and what were the barriers to dissemination? Several different types of evaluation methods and designs are needed to evaluate and understand dissemination (see Chapter 7).

Program monitoring (stage 6)

Beyond the dissemination stage, a **program of work** will become routinely **institutionalised** in the system (stage 6 in Figure 2.1 on page 24). The evaluation focus is directed towards supporting program management. These tasks include population-level monitoring of the outcome indicators of interest and continuing performance monitoring of the quality of program delivery. Although this stage is not considered in detail in this book, the assessment of 'quality' in health promotion has been given considerable attention in the recent past, and a number of guides and manuals have been produced to assist with this task (Brug et al. 2010). Methodologically, many of the tasks are essentially similar to process evaluation, described in Chapter 3.

As in any system, quality control in this stage requires close attention to ensure that implementation accords with established methods and standards of outcome. This also requires good monitoring of professional practice, combined with systems for routine measurement of health outcomes, risk factors and key determinants for health. This can help in monitoring the routine implementation of, or adherence to, an established program or policy that is delivered to all targeted people, settings or organisations.

Table 2.2 Case studies of research illustrating the stages in the model using different health promotion interventions

Stage of the model	Evaluation type	Principles underpinning case study	Case study
Stage 1: problem definition	Formative	International study of the prevalence of physical activity in 20 countries shows magnitude of public health problem and the need for public health action.	Bauman et al. (2009) described a 20-country study that used data from representative population **samples** to identify the proportion of adults that met the recommended guidelines for health-enhancing physical activity. The data identified countries that were more inactive and found subgroups where physical activity showed different social and socio-economic distribution.

Stage of the model	Evaluation type	Principles underpinning case study	Case study
Stage 2: solution generation	Formative	Behavioural research to identify the determinants of parents vaccinating their children—identified factors associated with vaccination; used individual level behavioural theory to identify factors.	Dube et al. (2012) carried out a large study in Canada to identify factors that determined what influenced parents vaccinated their young children against rotavirus (a cause of gastroenteritis). There were low rates of vaccination in this population and a need to identify why this was. Factors associated with vaccination over time were intention to immunise, beliefs about the vaccine and norms about vaccination in this population.
Stage 3: innovation testing	Impact/outcome evaluation	In low-to-middle-income countries, few community interventions evaluated to test efficacy/effectiveness of community-based interventions to reduce sexually transmitted infections (STIs).	Garcia et al. (2012) identified 20 communities in Peru, randomly allocated them to 10 intervention and 10 controls. Interventions comprised strengthened STI management, outreach to female sex workers and condom promotions. Results showed a non-significant decrease in STIs in intervention communities, but significant effects in subgroups, sex workers and younger women.
Stage 4: intervention demonstration	Impact/process	Replication of previously demonstrated effective smoking-prevention interventions 'in real-world conditions with usual classroom teachers'.	Nutbeam et al. (1993) conducted a controlled trial replicating the approach of previous research that had shown curriculum-based interventions to be effective in reducing youth smoking. The study trialled this approach in 'usual classroom conditions' in 39 schools in the UK. Schools were randomised to controls, with three interventions including family programs and curriculum changes. Rates of smoking adoption were similar across all four groups.

(continued)

Table 2.2 *continued*

Stage of the model	Evaluation type	Principles underpinning case study	Case study
Stage 5: intervention dissemination	Process	A series of studies titled 'Pool Cool' interventions in the USA targeted sun-protection practices at swimming pools; started with efficacy trials, moved to dissemination studies.	Escoffrey et al. (2009) described dissemination of Pool Cool program to more than 400 pools across the USA and described evaluation of dissemination; methods included implementation surveys, environmental audits, stakeholder and key informant surveys (to understand the processes of and barriers and facilitators of dissemination); also described in Glanz's (2011) summary paper.
Stage 6: program monitoring	Quality control monitoring and institutionalisation	Accepted prevention or health promotion intervention becoming routine in practice.	Examples in many countries would include routine childhood immunisation, banning smoking advertisements, providing free or low cost screening programs for at-risk age groups or populations (secondary prevention).

2.4   Quantitative and qualitative methods in program evaluation

Almost all of the research discussed in this chapter can be categorised as quantitative or qualitative. *Quantitative* methods are based on statistical principles and are heavily dependent on the quantifiable measurement of phenomena, particularly behaviours, and related psychological, social and environmental factors in such a way that they can be represented by numbers and statistically analysed (**observable phenomena**). This is especially useful for determining the outcome and effectiveness of a project or program. The challenge of developing reliable and valid measurements in health promotion is addressed in more detail in Chapter 5.

By contrast, *qualitative* research involves methods for examining, analysing and interpreting observations to discover underlying meanings of, and patterns in, relationships (**non-observable phenomena**). It is especially useful for understanding the process of implementation and explaining results obtained from quantitative research. Both quantitative and qualitative methods can contribute to each of the research stages described above. In many circumstances, they are synergistic and good-quality evaluation has components of both (Bartholomew et al. 2011).

Quantitative and qualitative methods in health promotion

Quantitative methods underpin much of the published research in health promotion. These methods are derived from approaches developed in epidemiology, quantitative behavioural and social sciences, statistics and demography. They focus on numeric data amenable to statistical analyses, which allow a researcher the opportunity to test ideas regarding the comparison of some attribute between groups, the assessment of changes over time or the association between two or more measures. In this approach, statistical testing (based on the probability of finding an observable difference) informs the researcher. A statement that the improvement over time is 'significant' means that it is unlikely to be due to chance or random variation alone (Chapter 5 gives more information on statistical tests). Quantitative methods are used where numeric data are available, and statistical tests performed to provide evidence in a traditional scientific method. Quantitative research follows a set of logical steps, from defining a testable research question, through the steps of research design, data collection, data analysis and interpretation, to finally reaching a conclusion.

As an example, it might be shown in the evaluation of project 1 on page 17 that people who attend the diabetes clinic make observable improvements in measures of dietary intake and measured body weight, compared to a group not attending the clinic, and these differences could be expressed statistically. Provided that the measures used are valid, this allows precise estimates of program effects to be made.

On the other hand, qualitative research methods have their historical roots in social sciences such as anthropology and political science. Methods include the use of focus groups (**structured discussions** with stakeholders or members of a target group) or directly learning from participating in or with target group members (ethnographic research or participant observation, sometimes called 'action research'). The processes of good qualitative research are the same as for quantitative research, moving through logical steps from identifying a clear research question to data collection, data analysis and interpretation. The data (information generated from this process) need to be analysed to give them structure, but are not directly amenable to statistical analysis. Thus, the original hypothesis (the idea that something may change following a health promotion intervention) is not proven or refuted through statistical analysis but rather through the interpretation of the researcher, based on the rules for good conduct of the particular type of qualitative research he or she is undertaking.

These qualitative methods are useful where information needs to be elicited from individuals or groups that are not already well-defined. For example, the women in project 2 on page 17 may have culturally specific beliefs about preventive care such as pap smears that will affect the likelihood of their participating in any program. These beliefs may be related to the gender of their health provider or to the perceived benefits of screening, and the health promoter may be unaware of these issues. Qualitative methods will be more efficient at identifying these beliefs or concerns, and this understanding could lead to the delivery of more effective programs and the development of more relevant measures to assess their relevance and effects. Information obtained from qualitative methods can often feed into the development and refinement of concepts and measures used in the quantitative phase of the evaluation.

Qualitative research methods may also be useful when asking community members to describe the:

- effects of a program;
- barriers to participation;
- strengths of program components.

In such circumstances, statistical data are not required. For example, in project 3 on page 18 a community-wide healthy nutrition program was proposed; here, stakeholder interviews with local restaurant owners could provide health promotion practitioners with useful information that enables identification of barriers and clear evaluation of effects. This qualitative information from restaurant owners could be obtained separately from any quantitative data obtained, either before the project is implemented to help with planning or after the intervention to provide additional information on why the intervention worked.

Using data-collection techniques that are less structured than those required for statistical analysis will allow a diversity of responses; it is a strength of qualitative methods that they can provide a broad range of both expected and unexpected information for program planning and assessment. This additional information collected following a program contributes to a better understanding of the program, to explain why it worked and to define which program elements were perceived as successful.

Despite this, qualitative research is frequently undervalued and underused. This is partly due to a values system that has evolved among some public health researchers which gives quantitative research high status and tends to devalue qualitative research, frequently referred to as 'soft' research. As a consequence, such methods may be either inappropriately applied or, when properly applied, inappropriately assessed.

As indicated above, although the methods may be different, qualitative research can be planned and executed using rigorous and careful methods. Identification of aims, selection and sampling of subjects, method of investigation and analysis of results can be as well defined and described in qualitative research as in quantitative research. This overview reveals that the best approach often uses both qualitative and quantitative methods. Neither are 'easy' methods.

> *Since health promotion programs can involve complex, multi-component interventions at many levels, it is often appropriate to observe the program from quantitative and qualitative perspectives.*

For example, it would be an indicator of success if the qualitative, semi-structured interviews of women indicated that the pap smear project (see example 2 in Section 2.1) was culturally acceptable and easily accessible. If the quantitative data indicated increased understanding of the role of cervical cancer screening, and increased pap smear attendance rates by women exposed to the intervention, then the quantitative data would corroborate (or *triangulate*) the qualitative findings. This so-called **triangulation** of information from different sources can be a very powerful tool in health promotion evaluation and is considered further in Chapter 6.

2.5 Formative, process and outcome evaluations

Figure 2.1 on page 24 also indicates the three key types of health promotion evaluation:
- formative evaluation;
- process evaluation;
- impact (or outcome) evaluation.

Formative evaluation is a set of activities designed to develop and pre-test project or program materials and methods, directed towards answering questions concerning relevance to identified health problems and the feasibility of different intervention methods (see Chapter 3 for more detail).

Process evaluation is a set of activities directed towards assessing progress in project/program implementation and recording the extent to which the program was implemented as planned and the circumstances in which it could be successfully and routinely reproduced.

Impact or outcome evaluation measures the effects that are predicted and defined during the planning stage of the program.

These form the central focus of the following chapters, building on Chapter 1, which introduced the idea of a continuous process of evaluation that starts when the program is first conceptualised and continues until after the program has finished. Evaluation may continue beyond the initial study, to assess the intervention as it is replicated and disseminated into other settings. In practice, time and attention are not necessarily divided equally among these evaluation types: pilot programs need mostly formative evaluation, while field studies in real-world settings tend to emphasise process evaluation. Health promotion projects or interventions set up as research studies, and large-scale, expensive program interventions, warrant greater investment in impact or outcome evaluation as well, which may require substantial support from research scientists.

The level of evaluation depends on the purposes of the intervention and also on its innovation. New programs that have never been tested should be assessed for their capacity to produce outcomes; existing programs that have been trialled elsewhere should be monitored to demonstrate that they are delivering programs of a consistent quality.

2.6   Summary

Evaluation of health promotion interventions is a complex enterprise and is often done poorly, using evaluation methods and measures inappropriate for the stage of an intervention's development. Many of the problems practitioners face in attempting to evaluate health promotion activity stem from unreasonable expectations of both the activity and the evaluation.

Not all programs need to be evaluated to the same level of intensity or using the same evaluation designs. The stages of evaluation shown in Figure 2.1 indicate how the evaluation question changes as a program evolves. The relative importance of formative, process and impact or outcome evaluations will vary as the research question and purpose of evaluation change. Each stage of developing, testing, replicating and disseminating a successful intervention requires a different evaluation design, choice of research methods and measure of success.

Both qualitative and quantitative research methods contribute to successful evaluations. In most cases, it is important to use evaluation designs that combine different research methodologies. The generation and use of a range of data and information sources generally provide more illuminating, relevant and sensitive evidence of effects than a single 'definitive' study. Process evaluation not only provides valuable information on how a program is implemented—as well as what activities occur, under what conditions, by whom and with what level of effort—but will also ensure that much more is learned and understood about success or failure in achieving defined outcomes. Through such insights, it is possible to identify the conditions that need to be created to achieve successful outcomes. Evaluations must be tailored to suit the activity and circumstances of individual programs: no single method can be 'right' for all programs.

References

Bartholomew LK, Parcel G & Kok G et al. 2011, *Planning Health Promotion Programs: An Intervention Mapping Approach*, Jossey-Bass, Wiley Publications, San Francisco, CA.

Bauman A, Bull F & Chey T et al. 2009, 'The International Prevalence Study on Physical Activity: results from 20 countries', *International Journal of Behavioral Nutrition and Physical Activity*, vol. 6.

Bauman AE, Sallis JF & Dzewaltowski DA et al. 2002, 'Towards a better understanding of the influences on physical activity: the role of determinants, correlates, causal variables, mediators, moderators and confounders', *American Journal of Preventative Medicine*, vol. 23 (2 Suppl), pp. 5–14.

Brug J, van Dale D & Lanting L et al. 2010, 'Towards evidence-based, quality-controlled health promotion: the Dutch recognition system for health promotion interventions', *Health Education Research*, vol. 25, no. 6, pp. 1100–6.

Dube E, Bettinger JA & Halperin B et al. 2012, 'Determinants of parents' decision to vaccinate their children against rotavirus: results of a longitudinal study', *Health Education Research*, vol. 27, no. 6, pp. 1069–80.

Escoffery C, Glanz K & Hall D et al. 2009, 'A multi-method process evaluation for a skin cancer prevention diffusion trial', *Evaluation and the Health Professions*, vol. 32, no. 2, pp. 184–203.

Garcia PJ, Holmes KK & Carcamo CP et al. 2012, 'Prevention of sexually transmitted infections in urban communities (Peru PREVEN): a multicomponent community-randomised controlled trial', *Lancet*, vol. 379, no. 9821, pp. 1120–8.

Glanz K 2011, 'Scale-up research: challenges and lessons learned from the Pool Cool diffusion trial', *Annals of Behavioral Medicine*, vol. 41, S153-S.

Nutbeam D, Harris E & Wise M 2010, *Theory in a Nutshell: A Practical Guide to Health Promotion Theories*, 3rd edn, McGraw-Hill, Sydney.

Nutbeam D, Macaskill P & Smith C et al. 1993, 'Evaluation of two school smoking education programmes under normal classroom conditions', *BMJ*, vol. 306, pp. 102–7.

3

Formative evaluation

Formative evaluation comprises the set of evaluation steps before launch or implementation of the intervention or program. Formative evaluation includes defining the need for the program, developing a 'best practice' intervention using available information, consulting with the target population and bringing these stages together into a program plan.

3.1 Formative evaluation: testing methods and materials before starting a project or program of work

Chapters 1 and 2 have shown that the evaluation cycle for a health promotion program starts with the generation of ideas to solve identified public health problems. These ideas may emerge from analysis of the problem or may be obtained from previously published scientific literature, colleagues or other sources. This initial idea needs to be tested and explored to determine the elements of a program that might be developed to solve the identified public health problem. This first stage of evaluation is described as *formative evaluation*, which is a set of activities designed to develop and pre-test program materials and methods. This is distinct from *process evaluation*, which is a set of activities directed towards assessing progress in program implementation (described in Chapter 4).

Formative evaluation occurs as part of program planning. Formative evaluation, according to the definition used in this book, always occurs before the intervention is launched; everything that occurs before the start (to the left of the launch in Figure 3.1) is 'formative'. This set of activities is concerned with the stages from initial concept, through development, testing and refinement to the final planned intervention.

In considering program planning in Chapter 1, we recognised that, despite the best intentions, in many cases practitioners find themselves under pressure to deliver a program quickly and may neglect to consider the preparatory work required before the program starts. These examples

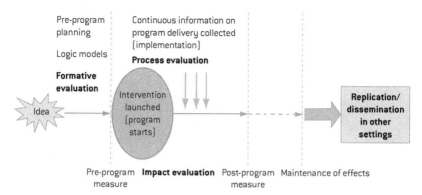

Figure 3.1 Stages showing formative, process and impact/outcome evaluations

demonstrate how important formative evaluation can be to the development of a relevant and appropriate program.

Formative evaluation would normally occur in consultation with stakeholders and/or with members of the population that is the target for an intervention. Through this process, the key methods and materials that form an intervention are identified. Formative evaluation uses a diverse range of quantitative and qualitative methods to define and develop the elements likely to be effective in the program.

Several categories of activities fall into the category of formative evaluation. These include:

1.   Reviewing the problem and assessing previous efforts to address it. This is often the initial step in formative evaluation, and consists of identifying that the problem is of sufficient magnitude and importance in the target population or community to warrant public health approaches. All sources of community and population data can be used here, including previous research, existing population surveys and routine data collections. In addition, non-health data, such as information about income, socioeconomic deprivation, cultural groups, and facilities and resources in the community can all contribute to planning an intervention.

The next step is the process of reviewing the literature to assess the impact of similar interventions in similar settings, or to identify research summarising intervention effects across studies, or describing 'best practice' in a particular intervention area (see Box 3.1 on page 40 and also Chapter 8 for a discussion of evidence summaries and 'systematic reviews').

Box 3.1 The role of systematic reviews in identifying 'best practice'

One of the stages in formative evaluation is finding out what effective programs have been tried in other places and settings. This involves identifying what have others done, and what is considered 'best practice' for an intervention or project. Best practice is derived from both formal scientific evidence reviews and practice-based reports (Green et al. 2009), but the former is typically the starting point in program planning.

Scientific reviews can be narrative (descriptive), systematic or formal statistical pooling of intervention effects (meta-analyses). Systematic reviews are often used in assessing health promotion program evidence. They compare interventions addressing the same issue, and have standard methods and inclusion criteria before a subset of studies is compared. The summary of evidence can help to:

1. identify whether there are sufficient papers in a field to make a judgment;
2. indicate which intervention approaches might be most effective in achieving outcomes.

Systematic reviews can assess and summarise different elements in program evaluation. They can assess program effectiveness in community (or other) settings (Shahab & McEwen 2009); economic outcomes (van Dongen et al. 2011); intervention characteristics (Laplante 2011); recruitment to interventions (Foster et al. 2011); and interventions in low-to-middle-income countries (Hall 2011, Vindigni et al. 2009). They can also summarise the use of evidence by policy-makers (Orton et al. 2011).

2. Understanding the target population or community.
   Qualitative and quantitative techniques are used to identify information about the community, often using a participatory planning approach, engaging with the community to plan a health promotion program. This kind of formative evaluation identifies what issues people have surrounding a health problem, what barriers and facilitators might exist, and what types of solutions the community members would support. In addition, this information gathering may identify subgroups that might benefit more from an intervention, and opportunities and community resources that might be deployed to assist an intervention. The methods include consultation with key stakeholders and/or community members, often using small-group discussions, focus groups, semi-structured interviews and prioritisation techniques for choosing among alternatives.

3. Pre-testing intervention methods and materials.
   Formative evaluation is also concerned with pilot testing of interventions or intervention materials with samples of the target audience. For example, printed resources or specific messages can be tested and compared in groups similar to the target audience. Formative evaluation can be used to test alternative approaches or

materials in small groups, to identify preferences for delivery and scope of interventions. These pilot studies can assess the feasibility of the proposed intervention, to assess whether it is thought acceptable and potentially useful for the proposed target population. Pilot studies can use rigorous scientific designs and can even be randomised trials (see Chapter 5), but in small samples and with the purpose of identifying likely effective interventions to be applied to much larger samples and to whole populations.

4. Using formative evaluation for program planning.
    Program planning is also part of the work required before implementing an intervention. An example of program planning, the development of a logic model, was described in Chapter 2. Other planning techniques, such as intervention mapping (IM), also are part of the pre-program work to define and describe the proposed program and its theoretical underpinnings.

    The overall purposes of formative evaluation are to prepare the ground for delivering an intevention that is the best possible, will be most acceptable to the community or target population and will be likely to improve health and meet community needs closely. Formative evaluation can assess whether a program is ready for evaluation (this is known as 'evaluability assessment'). The results of formative evaluation do not imply that a guaranteed program will follow; it is a step in program assessment and development and, if further intervention development may be required as the next action, to produce a program likely to be effective or acceptable. Too often health promotion program funding cycles have limited time frames, and the lack of feasibility or promise is ignored in the rush to implement 'a program', although formative evaluation suggests it will be ineffective.

Table 3.1 on pages 43–5 provides illustrative case studies of health promotion interventions that used different types of formative evaluation to test interventions, shape intervention methods and develop support materials and program elements. These case studies illustrate formative evaluation in large-scale community trials as well as the developmental work that underpins smaller health promotion programs. They also illustrate the range of possible research methods and settings for formative evaluation.

Undertaking formative evaluation will significantly determine the likelihood of subsequent success and failure as well as building a sound basis for the chosen process and outcome evaluation.

The first set of examples show the use of formative evaluation to understand the issues and the target population. Researchers have identified the magnitude and correlates or determinants of many health promotion problems, and a review of the literature identifies some possible starting points for intervention planning. Qualitative methods can uncover cultural and national differences in the ways problems are perceived or solved (Verbestel et al. 2011). Systematic or narrative reviews of published studies should be sought, as evidence for program effectiveness may already exist (see Box 3.1 on page 40).

The next set of studies are exemplars of formative evaluation to understand the target population. Davies et al. (2009) describe the development of a parenting and social support program targeting the particular needs identified for mothers of children with HIV. Community consultation and participation are important in developing relevant programs in communities (Doorenbos et al. 2011). Formative evaluation is common in designing mass media messages, mass campaigns and social marketing interventions, and formative research establishes communication goals, and identifies simple relevant messages targeting beliefs and behaviours in specific target groups. Table 3.1 on pages 43–5 shows some examples of message development around use of illicit drugs and adolescent smoking cessation (Keijseras 2008, Latimer et al. 2012). Partnerships with target group members are essential to develop appropriate and acceptable messages, especially around sensitive issues such as illicit drug use, or in culturally or socially defined subgroups. These formative studies often include a mix of qualitative and quantitative evaluation methods (Riekert et al. 2011).

Sometimes this formative evaluation will expose differences in the interpretation of priorities for action between 'experts' or researchers compared to the target group.

> *Understanding the needs of the target audience, and using formative research to develop appropriate and accepted intervention methods and materials, are an essential first step in designing an effective intervention. Involving stakeholders and funders at this formative stage will also make a sustainable intervention more likely.*

Researchers also use formative evaluation to test pilot interventions. Here, small sample randomised trials may be conducted, using volunteers, to assess if an intervention is likely to work and to choose the most efficacious among alternative versions of an intervention (Table 3.1). For example,

Table 3.1 Examples of the uses of formative evaluation in health promotion

Type of formative evaluation	Author (year)	Research methods used	Use of formative evaluation results
1. Reviewing the problem and previous efforts to address it			
Identify prevalence and correlates of physical activity	Bauman et al. (2012)	Review of >600 studies that described social, environmental and individual factors associated with physical activity in adults and children.	Identify the consistency of correlates and determinant factors in high- and middle-income countries—and therefore their usefulness in intervention planning.
Large-scale obesity prevention to address children (in Europe)	Verbestel et al. (2011)	Focus groups/discussions with different centres, understanding context differences, adaptation.	Identifies differences needed in implementing childhood obesity programs in different countries.
Systematic reviews	See Box 3.1—identify if there are reviews or summaries of interventions in the area of interest.		
2. Understanding the target population or community			
Formative development of parenting and support program	Davies et al. (2009)	Targeting mothers with HIV. Qualitative methods (focus groups, interviews).	Identified salient program components most relevant to consumers.
Program to develop Cancer Control Telehealth Network (Indigenous Americans)	Doorenbos et al. (2011)	Community participation and consultation with health workers and consumers regarding telehealth interventions.	Identified effective elements of a cancer control network, which was then implemented.
Large-scale program to reduce illicit drug harms (cocaine imports)	Keijsers et al. (2008)	Illicit-drug monitoring system (quantitative) and Delphi technique (qualitative).	Identified ways of portraying warning messages, mutual understanding with target groups, improvements to monitoring.
Message development and testing (for adolescent-targeted smoking cessation)	Latimer et al. (2012)	Message testing (quasi-experimental crossover design testing message preferences, content and message framing).	Provided direction for adolescent smoking-cessation messages and video production; identified preference for peer-led cessation interventions.

[continued]

Table 3.1 *continued*

Type of formative evaluation	Author (year)	Research methods used	Use of formative evaluation results
Develop intervention for asthma therapy adherence among African-American adolescents	Riekert et al. (2011)	Assess feasibility of motivational interviewing for asthma education (qualitative, and then piloting intervention).	Suggests motivational interviewing is feasible for adolescents with asthma.
3. Pre-testing intervention methods and materials			
Testing acceptability of program for refugee women	De Stephano et al. (2010)	Low-literacy setting for testing the acceptability of prenatal education videos.	Video format acceptable to refugee women, found them helpful and culturally tailored for antenatal clinic setting.
Pilot of intervention (youth smokers)	Abroms et al. (2008)	Pilot randomised controlled testing (RCT) of efficacy of different interventions targeting youth smoking.	Identified which intervention to use among different options.
Pilot of smoking in pregnancy intervention, with community consultation	Bryce (2009)	Action research, to reduce smoking in young women in pregnancy.	Demonstrated feasibility for antenatal services and consumers (context).
Pilot of children's physical-activity program	Jurg et al. (2008)	Pilot intervention, development of health promotion outcomes ('social action', and healthy public policy, leading to 'health literacy').	Development of intervention and of health promotion and intermediate measures, and improved understanding of implementation challenges.
4. Using formative evaluation for program planning			
HIV-prevention intervention mapping (IM), a method of program planning	Corbie-Smith et al. (2012)	IM carried out with community participation to develop interventions targeting HIV prevention.	Developed multi-generational HIV-prevention programs; used IM to plan and sequence program components.

IM to develop adolescent smoking intervention	Dalum et al. (2012)	IM used to develop theory-based intervention alongside needs assessment.	Identified behavioural journalism and motivational interviewing as promising strategies in this target group.
IM for Dutch adolescent physical-activity program development	Prins et al. (2010)	IM to define program objectives, theory used, plan for pre-testing.	Developed appropriate computer-tailored interventions targeting Dutch youth.
Using logic models for planning physical-activity programs in Brazil	Ribeiro (2010)	Twelve-month process of developing logic model for a community intervention on physical activity.	Logic model helped to frame evaluation questions, identified measures needed and partnerships required for community action.
Using logic models to plan a national mass-media campaign in the USA	Huhman et al. (2004)	Identified information available, planned media campaigns, community infrastructure needs.	Logic model described outcomes at multiple levels, including community indicators.
Logic models for a community youth mental-health program in Beirut	Afifi et al. (2011)	Used community consultation with parents and adolescents, teachers.	Designed program targeting social-network development, school policies, civic engagement by adolescents to improve mental health.

piloting of interventions can compare interventions with control groups in small samples, or compare alternate interventions to assess which might work best in a scaled-up intervention (Abroms et al. 2008). De Stephano et al. (2010) tested the acceptability of health promotion resources and materials with a sample of low-literacy refugee women, and Bryce demonstrated the feasibility of a new antenatal smoking program to be introduced into a health service. Jurg (2008) piloted a children's physical-activity intervention and developed a range of intermediate outcome measures for use in a larger study (Table 3.1).

Examples of program planning through IM and logic models are illustrated at the end of Table 3.1. The study by Corbie-Smith et al. (2010) describes the planning of multi-generational HIV-prevention programs; Dalum et al. (2012) use IM to plan adolescent smoking interventions; Prins et al. (2010) also use IM to describe theory and program objectives for an adolescent physical-activity intervention. Formative evaluation can also be used to test the use of theories relevant to health promotion. For further information on theories used in health promotion, refer to the companion publication, *Theory in a Nutshell* (Nutbeam et al. 2010). Three examples of the use of logic models are shown, for planning a community intervention in Brazil (Ribeiro 2010), for planning a national mass-media campaign (Huhman et al. 2004) and for developing a youth mental-health program in Lebanon (Afifi et al. 2011).

'Formative research' in the literature and 'process evaluation' in this book

Some researchers use the term 'formative evaluation' to describe 'program improvement', as well as program development. In this book, assessing 'program improvement during delivery' is considered part of 'process evaluation', as it occurs after the start or launch of the intervention (Figure 3.1). For example, a 'formative evaluation' of a walking program in England (Milton et al. 2011) assessed delivery of the intervention through interviews with staff to improve the program; since these occurred after the start of the program, and helped in developing an understanding of program implementation, this would be considered 'process evaluation' by definition in this book. Similarly, 'formative evaluation to increase vaccination rates' (Wallace & LeGro 2008) collected quantitative and qualitative information during the intervention, to understand it and improve it; again, because this took place during the implementation phase, our model considers it 'process evaluation'. Use of Figure 3.1 can resolve the issue whether a set of evaluation tasks should be described as 'formative' or 'process', based on when the evaluation information was collected.

3.2 Formative evaluation for different types of health promotion intervention

Formative evaluation applies to many contexts and types of intervention. Behavioural researchers, planning individual behaviour change interventions, have specific needs for formative studies. Key formative tasks are identifying and validating behavioural measures of intermediate variables and of program outcomes, testing the interventions in pilot studies, and assessing program feasibility (Baranowski et al. 2009). This is specific to planning tightly controlled interventions for behaviour change, but demonstrates the need for formative evaluation at all levels and types of health promotion program.

Mass media campaigns use formative evaluation to develop and test concepts and messages. Other media, resources and styles of individually focused health promotion intervention delivery can also be pre-tested in formative studies. Environmental and policy interventions use formative research to develop measures that might indicate success in influencing the physical or social environment, measuring community partnership and social capital, and testing the community acceptability of innovative infrastructure changes.

Formative evaluation is also useful in large-scale, multi-component health promotion programs. Here, formative evaluation might include stakeholder consultations to identify context differences for implementation and a range of 'minimal intervention' materials that might be used across a wide range of settings. Even when programs are scaled up to reach larger populations, formative evaluation can assess the conditions for increasing the reach of the intervention, through formative research with stakeholders and policy-makers. This indicates that formative evaluation can and should occur prior to implementing an efficacy study (stage 3 in Figure 2.1 on page 24) or prior to a replication or dissemination study (stages 4 and 5 in Figure 2.1). An example of formative research for dissemination can be found in O'Hara (2013).

3.3 Summary

Despite practitioners' best intentions, they are often under pressure to deliver a program quickly and may neglect to consider the required preparatory (formative) work before the start of a program. Although it will not always be possible to conduct comprehensive formative evaluation, this is an essential first step in the evaluation process. Undertaking formative evaluation will affect the likelihood of subsequent success or failure, as well as building a sound basis for subsequent process and outcome evaluation.

Using qualitative and quantitative research methods, formative evaluation is the first step towards testing the underlying need for a program and ascertaining its relevance to the target population. Formative evaluation provides program planners with information to use in assessing how the intervention might work, and provides a roadmap for implementation. It helps to test an intervention's feasibility and to predict the likely community responses to proposed activities. In practical terms, formative evaluation enables the development of the best possible intervention, using the most relevant methods and materials.

References

Abroms LC, Windsor R & Simons-Morton B 2008, 'Getting young adults to quit smoking: a formative evaluation of the X-Pack Program', *Nicotine and Tobacco Research*, vol. 10, no. 1, pp. 27–33.

Afifi RA, Makhoul J & Hajj T et al. 2011, 'Developing a logic model for youth mental health: participatory research with a refugee community in Beirut', *Health Policy Plan*, vol. 26, no. 6, pp. 508–17.

Baranowski T, Cerin E & Baranowski J 2009, 'Steps in the design, development and formative evaluation of obesity prevention-related behavior change trials', *International Journal of Behavioral Nutrition and Physical Activity*, vol. 21, no. 6, p. 6.

Bauman AE, Reis RS & Sallis JF et al. 2012, 'Correlates of physical activity: why are some people physically active and others not?' *Lancet*, vol. 21, no. 380(9838), pp. 258–71.

Corbie-Smith G, Akers A & Blumenthal C et al. 2010, 'Intervention mapping as a participatory approach to developing an HIV prevention intervention in rural African American communities', *AIDS Education and Prevention*, vol. 22, no. 3, pp. 184–202.

Dalum P, Schaalma H & Kok G 2012, 'The development of an adolescent smoking cessation intervention: an intervention mapping approach to planning', *Health Education Research*, vol. 27, no. 1, pp. 172–81.

Davies SL, Horton TV & Williams AG et al. 2009, 'MOMS: formative evaluation and subsequent intervention for mothers living with HIV', *AIDS Care: Psychological and Socio-Medical Aspects of AIDS/HIV*, vol. 21, no. 5, pp. 552–60.

De Stephano CC, Flynn PM & Brost BC 2010, 'Somali prenatal education video use in a United States obstetric clinic: a formative evaluation of acceptability', *Patient Education and Counseling*, vol. 81, no. 1, pp. 137–41.

Doorenbos AZ, Demiris G & Towle C et al. 2011, 'Developing the native people for Cancer Control Telehealth Network', *Telemedicine and E-Health*, vol. 17, no. 1, pp. 30–4.

Foster CE, Brennan G & Matthews A et al. 2011, 'Recruiting participants to walking intervention studies: a systematic review', *International Journal of Behavioral Nutrition and Physical Activity*, vol. 15, no. 8, p. 137.

Green LW, Ottoson JM & Garcia C 2009, 'Diffusion theory and knowledge dissemination, utilization, and integration in public health', *Annual Review of Public Health*, vol. 30, pp. 151–74.

Hall J 2011, 'Effective community-based interventions to improve exclusive breast feeding at four to six months in low- and low-to-middle-income countries: a systematic review of randomised controlled trials', *Midwifery*, vol. 27, no. 4, pp. 497–502.

Huhman M, Heitzler C & Wong F 2004, 'The VERB campaign logic model: a tool for planning and evaluation', *Preventing Chronic Disease*, vol. 1, no. 3 (July), A11.

Jurg ME, De Meij JSB & Van der Wal MF et al. 2008, 'Using health promotion outcomes in formative evaluation studies to predict success factors in interventions: an application to an intervention for promoting physical activity in Dutch children (JUMP-in)', *Health Promotion International*, vol. 23, no. 3, pp. 231–9.

Keijsers L, Bossong MG & Waarlo AJ 2008, 'Participatory evaluation of a Dutch warning campaign for substance-users', *Health Risk and Society*, vol. 10, no. 3, pp. 283–95.

Laplante C & Peng W 2011, 'A systematic review of e-health interventions for physical activity: an analysis of study design, intervention characteristics, and outcomes', *Telemedicine and E-Health*, vol. 17, no. 7, pp. 509–23.

Latimer AE, Krishnan-Sarin S & Cavallo DA et al. 2012, 'Targeted smoking cessation messages for adolescents', *Journal of Adolescent Health*, vol. 50, no. 1, pp. 47–53.

Milton K, Kelly P & Bull F et al. 2011, 'A formative evaluation of a family-based walking intervention: Furness Families Walk4Life', *BMC Public Health*, vol. 2, no. 11, p. 614.

Nutbeam D, Harris E & Wise M 2010, *Theory in a Nutshell: A Practical Guide to Health Promotion Theories*, 3rd edn, McGraw-Hill, Sydney.

O'Hara BJ, Phongsavan P & King L et al. 2013, 'Translational formative evaluation: critical in up-scaling public health programmes', *Health Promotion International* (28 April: epub prior to print publication).

Orton L, Lloyd-Williams F & Taylor-Robinson D et al. 2011, 'The use of research evidence in public health decision making processes: systematic review', *PLoS One*, vol. 6, no. 7, e21704.

Prins RG, van Empelen P & Beenackers MA et al. 2010, 'Systematic development of the YouRAction program, a computer-tailored physical activity promotion intervention for Dutch adolescents, targeting personal motivations and environmental opportunities', *BMC Public Health*, vol. 11, no. 10, p. 474.

Ribeiro IC, Torres A & Parra DC et al. 2010, 'Using logic models as iterative tools for planning and evaluating physical activity promotion programs in Curitiba, Brazil', *Journal of Physical Activity and Health*, vol. 7, S155-S62.

Riekert KA, Borrelli B & Bilderback A et al. 2011, 'The development of a motivational interviewing intervention to promote medication adherence among inner-city, African-American adolescents with asthma', *Patient Education and Counseling*, vol. 82, no. 1, pp. 117–22.

Shahab, L & McEwen, A 2009, 'Online support for smoking cessation: a systematic review of the literature', *Addiction*, vol. 4, no. 11, pp. 1792–804.

van Dongen JM, Proper KI & van Wier MF et al. 2011, 'Systematic review on the financial return of worksite health promotion programs aimed at improving nutrition and/or increasing physical activity', *Obesity Reviews*, vol. 12, no. 12, pp. 1031–49.

Verbestel V, De Henauw S & Maes L et al. 2011, 'Using the intervention mapping protocol to develop a community-based intervention for the prevention of childhood obesity in a multi-centre European project: the IDEFICS intervention', *International Journal of Behavioral Nutrition and Physical Activity*, vol. 1, no. 8 (August), p. 82.

Vindigni SM, Riley PL & Jhung M 2011, 'Systematic review: handwashing behaviour in low-to-middle-income countries: outcome measures and behaviour maintenance', *Tropical Medicine and International Health*, vol. 16, no. 4, pp. 466–77.

Wallace CM & Legro MW 2008, 'Using formative evaluation in an implementation project to increase vaccination rates in high-risk veterans: QUERI Series', *Implementation Science*, vol. 22, no. 3, p. 22.

4

Process evaluation

Process evaluation comprises the set of activities surrounding program or intervention implementation, acceptance and population reach. It describes how the program is carried out in practice, and how it may be implemented differently in diverse environments. Process evaluation helps to understand how the program was delivered and why it did or did not achieve its anticipated outcomes.

4.1 Assessing the implementation of health promotion projects and programs

Process evaluation is a set of activities directed towards assessing progress in the implementation of a project or program. Process evaluation describes and explains what happens once the project or program has started (see Chapter 3, Figure 3.1), and contributes to an understanding of how and why interventions work and which elements contribute to their effectiveness. Process evaluation can also help explain modest or negligible effects (why interventions do *not* work). Process evaluation starts when the definitive intervention is launched or initiated following planning and formative evaluation. It is often conducted concurrently with *impact* evaluation (see Figure 3.1). Planning for process evaluation occurs before the intervention starts, and needs to be well established and integrated into intervention maps (IM) or logic models (for more detail on these, see Chapter 3).

It follows that a broad range of activities comprise process evaluation. Process evaluation identifies whether target groups were exposed to, and participated in, the intervention and whether stakeholders and partners engaged with it. It also encompasses assessment of the short-term impact of an intervention: the *health promotion outcomes* (described in Chapter 2, Figure 2.1). The achievement of these outcomes is part of the 'process' of achieving the longer term outcomes that are described in Chapter 1.

> *The aims of process evaluation are to understand how the program worked, what happened in 'real life' and how people reacted to it.*

These are intervening steps in the processes of change. Understanding these processes is the most fundamental aspect of any health promotion program evaluation. It is simply unrealistic to expect a program to succeed if it has not reached the target groups, involved the appropriate stakeholders or engaged with the community as intended. It is an integral and explanatory part of program evaluation (stage 3, shown in Figure 2.1, Chapter 2) to assess whether the different program elements were delivered as intended. It is also an essential part of stage 4 studies of program reproducibility (see Figure 2.1). Here, the evidence for program effectiveness is acknowledged through earlier studies, and the process of assessing the reach, adoption and utilisation of the program is assessed.

Process evaluation occurs across all stages of building evidence in Figure 2.1. Process evaluation is an important part of intervention testing to assess effectiveness or efficacy. It is also used to understand the replication and dissemination of programs to wider settings (stages 4 and 5, shown in Figure 2.1), to identify whether the effective parts of the program, for example, adherence to an intervention curriculum, are maintained when the program has been disseminated in multiple field settings. For example, an evidence-based health promotion program may be developed and trialled in one set of schools, but when it is implemented across a state or region in many schools, it will inevitably undergo some local adaptation. Monitoring how the program is implemented in the many schools is critical to understanding whether dissemination was effective. Recording these adaptations and modifications to intervention delivery in the field, and analysing their potential impact on the program's effectiveness, are core to an evaluation of the successful dissemination of a program.

Disappointingly, process evaluation is often not carried out, or is not conducted to a high standard. For understandable reasons (such as pressure to demonstrate results), the resources available for evaluation are often exclusively channelled into outcome assessment. This means that often we may not know how well a program was implemented, and consequently may not be able to explain why it was successful or unsuccessful in achieving predetermined outcomes. This knowledge is useful for practitioners. If a program has been successful, good process evaluation will identify how it worked and some of the mechanisms through which successful programs operate. Alternatively, if a program fails to achieve predetermined outcomes, process evaluation can help to identify the potential causes of that failure and support subsequent modification to make future success more likely.

Monitoring program implementation is of importance to managers. It is a quality-assurance tool, providing rapid feedback on the quality and integrity of the implementation and identifying possible improvements in program delivery. Process evaluation can also identify whether resources were adequate for implementation, and whether the program could be repeated elsewhere or whether different investments, different population group targeting or alternative programs should be considered.

Process evaluation can include a broad range of methods and measurements, but there are some more common elements:

- Exposure: assessing whether participants were aware of the issue being addressed, received the program or were aware of the messages being communicated.

- Participation: identifying how well individuals, relevant groups and organisations were recruited to the program (for more on systematic review of recruitment, see Foster et al. 2011). This could include the recruitment of people with a defined health problem, community members or even recruitment of organisations such as schools or work sites, partner agencies and non-government organisations (NGOs). Rates of participation may help to explain subsequent effects; low participation may lead to poorer results or to selection effects that influence the program (see Chapter 5); generally, high participation and attendance at most program sessions make successful outcomes more likely.

- Delivery: assessing whether or not the program was delivered using the methods and materials as designed (known as *program fidelity*). Systematic use of a logic model can provide a good reference point for the assessment of program delivery.

- Program satisfaction and usage: assessment of program satisfaction and usage might look at the extent to which participants used the resources, attended classes or participated in community activities in the way that was intended, and whether they found these program elements to be relevant and useful to their needs (perceived relevance and intended use of the program are much more important than 'program satisfaction', which is subject to social desirability bias, especially if asked immediately after a program by those who delivered the program).

- Context: examining reasons why the program was implemented as it was. This would include examination of the context in which the program was implemented, taking into account such variables as social influences, community opinion, economic factors, climate and changes in the physical environment, all of which may have an impact on participation and delivery. Variations from the original protocol and adaptation of the intervention to local conditions are common in health promotion programs. Systematic recording of methods and materials used in delivering an intervention will help explain subsequent outcomes.

4.2 Methods for conducting process evaluation

Table 4.1 provides some examples of practical steps in conducting real-world process evaluation. These are things that practitioners can do and information that can be collected during an intervention as a part of process evaluation. Most of these activities involve collecting information: keeping records of program activity, conducting audits of program attendance and participation, and keeping structured records of stakeholder engagement. There are no fixed rules on which intervention elements to monitor, but all clearly articulated components of an IM or logic model should be monitored.

Process evaluation uses both quantitative and qualitative methods, in what can be described as a 'mixed methods' evaluation. Quantitative data may comprise surveys or other instruments, and simple counts may comprise numerical data, for example, about usage of resources or attendance at events, or measures of community coalitions and partnership formation.

Researchers often wish to quantify the amount of the program that was delivered as intended (program *exposure*), the reach of the program (*proportion* of the eligible target group that participates) and the extent to which the program was delivered as intended (the *fidelity* of program delivery). For example, if half the target group only attended two out of four classes and one-fifth attended none, then 'dose of intervention received' can be accurately described, and outcomes examined, in relation to the amount of program exposure.

The reach of the program is important for understanding 'generalisability', a measure of how far the program participants represent the general population. Low reach may imply that selected volunteers attended programs, and the observed effects may be confined to motivated groups or sub-populations. Estimates of program reach are important from a population health perspective, especially to identify if any subgroups were less likely to attend. These are often disadvantaged or marginalised subgroups, and it is essential to quantify their participation because additional services or different programs may be required to meet their needs.

Sometimes satisfaction surveys are used as part of process evaluation, but these often suffer from social desirability bias, with many people keen

Table 4.1 Practical tasks in carrying out process evaluation tasks

Process evaluation tasks	Examples of what practitioners could actually do
Exposure to the intervention/ elements of the intervention	■ Assess 'exposure' to the intervention by quantitative survey or by qualitative focused discussions or interviews with samples of the target group or stakeholders to identify their level of awareness of the program, and whether they were exposed to it, recognised it or engaged with it. From the practitioner perspective, failure to achieve understanding and recognition at this most basic level will have a fundamental impact on subsequent participation.
Participation (describing intervention participation rates); these include measures of 'recruitment' to the program and 'reach into a population', program satisfaction	■ Identify how many people were expected to participate; count numbers actually attending each session or component (this is a measure of the **representativeness** of participants; if those in the program are different to the whole population from which they were drawn, then the intervention has a 'selected' (biased) sample of participants). ■ Keep a record of the proportion who attended all sessions or events. How many attended only some sessions, or none? Document if there were specific subgroups who did not attend but were expected (for example, people without cars, people from specific cultural or language groups, frail elderly adults with reduced mobility and so on). ■ Measure program satisfaction and, even more importantly, engagement with and use of the intervention materials by program participants, and/or assess perceptions about the program among stakeholders. ■ Monitor and document staff time, engagement (for example, did it take longer to run the program in different contexts?).
Delivery of the intervention, or assessing scaling-up of the intervention to larger population	■ Record and monitor the number of sessions delivered, the location and completeness of program delivery at different sites. Record ways in which program delivery differed at different sites; this is assessing program 'fidelity' (was the program delivered in exactly the way it was intended; document any adaptations made to deliver the program).
Context of the intervention (this is about describing the different settings and contexts in which programs are delivered)	■ Keep a log of problems in the delivery of the intervention, difficulties experienced, barriers to implementation reported by staff. ■ Interview a sample of staff, stakeholders and participants regarding the environmental and social reasons, costs or other factors that influenced the implementation of the intervention. ■ Record ways in which the program was delivered differently in different settings (for example, what happened when support materials were not available as required, or program materials were delivered to a target population in a way that was different to what was planned?).

to please the program staff and unwilling to divulge program problems and difficulties. Such surveys will often produce 'positive results', as participants report that they 'liked the program' and appreciated the efforts of those who delivered it. Unless this type of survey is very carefully conducted, it will not provide quality information on the process of implementation.

In order to identify the strengths and weaknesses of projects, qualitative methods are often useful. Semi-structured interviews or focus groups with participants and, ideally, some non-participants can identify perceptions of an intervention, or problems with access, language or program complexity that were not previously recognised. This can inform health promotion practitioners of issues *during the project*, enabling them to take corrective action. Similarly, qualitative assessment of large-scale programs can be informative to identify a lack of component reach or resources, and differential implementation of program elements in different settings.

Table 4.2 shows examples of published studies that use process evaluation in different ways and in different settings. This not a comprehensive list of all uses of process evaluation, but does illustrate some common principles.

The first set of process evaluation studies in Table 4.2 shows examples of process evaluation that describe intervention reach and exposure to intervention messages or resources, and report program feasibility and participant satisfaction with the intervention. Examples are drawn from the contexts of HIV prevention (Hargreaves et al. 2010), workplace interventions and health risk appraisals (Colkesen et al. 2011), injury prevention in schools (Collard et al. 2010) and media campaigns on quitting smoking (Hong et al. 2008). One study in India reports comprehensive process evaluation measures, but cautions against program satisfaction measures because of social desirability bias, the likelihood of participants to report mostly 'positive' features of a program (Goenka et al. 2010).

The second set of examples describes some measures used in process evaluation, including indicators of partnership development and engagement (Cheadle et al. 2008). Common themes also occur across projects as process indicators of successful implementation, including community participation and involvement (Eni & Rowe 2011, Rath et al. 2010). Process evaluations use multiple research methods, but qualitative methods are commonplace, including focus group discussions, interviews and observations.

The next group of process evaluations focuses on delivery and variation in implementation in diverse contexts (Mukoma et al. 2009, Perez et al. 2011, Singh et al. 2009). In addition, they show similar factors associated with implementation, including resources, training and local leadership. One project used process measures to understand why a falls-prevention trial was ineffective (Logghe et al. 2011), a very important but under-used form of process evaluation. This use of process evaluation to understand how programs work and why they may fail can also be assessed using complex and quantitative methods. These are discussed in Box 4.1 on page 60.

The last set of examples in Table 4.2 shows process evaluation at later stages in the evidence generation process (see also Chapter 2, Figure 2.1). Here, examples of process evaluation illustrate factors associated with the large-scale implementation of a smoking-prevention program (English et al. 2010), and in replication and dissemination studies (Griffin et al. 2010, Escoffrey et al. 2008), assessing the implementation of already effective programs delivered in multiple settings across a wide region.

Table 4.2 Examples of process evaluation (PE)

Program description (place)	Author (year)	Types of PE used	Usefulness of PE for the program
Process evaluation: exposure to intervention, reported program satisfaction, feasibility			
Micro-finance intervention for HIV prevention (rural South Africa)	Hargreaves et al. (2010)	Assessed feasibility and acceptability of micro-finance; measures of program attendance; questionnaires and focus group discussions.	Found micro-finance to be feasible and acceptable for most clients; some barriers identified useful for future programs.
Workplace web-intervention and health-risk appraisal	Colkesen et al. (2011)	Identifies characteristics of participants in health-risk appraisals.	Relevant to planning workplace health promotion (HP) intervention, identifying 'motivated' healthier people who were likely to participate.
Process evaluation of a program to reduce injuries in schools	Collard et al. (2010)	Documented participation rate (reach) at school and pupil levels; described implementation 'as intended' (*fidelity*) documented by teachers' logs.	Provides framework for using several types of PE to monitor injury-prevention program.
PE of school-based media campaign for students to quit smoking (USA)	Hong et al. (2008)	Assessed campaign reach, exposure, response to and perceptions of the media messages to quit smoking.	Reported awareness, whether students liked the messages, and whether they used the messages to quit smoking.

(*continued*)

Table 4.2 *continued*

Program description (place)	Author (year)	Types of PE used	Usefulness of PE for the program
Tobacco prevention program in schools (India)	Goenka et al. (2010)	Mixed-methods PE assessed; dose of intervention received; student numbers participating; teacher training.	Limitations in some PE measures due to social desirability bias in reporting; peer-led components seemed effective.
Process evaluation: participation, reach, understanding program effects			
Process evaluation of local health department partnerships (California)	Cheadle et al. (2008)	QA; assessing capacity-building; policy change; developed indicators of increased partnerships; shared planning and community engagement.	PE measured partnerships and commitment as intermediate factors in community program implementation. Demonstrates PE assessed at the organisational level.
Parenting program in first nations (Canada)	Eni & Rowe (2011)	65 open-ended, semi-structured interviews in 13 communities.	Qualitative themes emerged as supportive factors or barriers to intervention implementation: social support, community support, social disadvantage.
Maternal/ child health intervention (India)	Rath et al. (2010)	Part of a cluster randomised trial of community mobilisation and education, capacity-building for women.	Implementation influenced by factors: program acceptability, participatory approaches, community involvement and active recruitment.
Process evaluation: delivery, context			
Process evaluation of mosquito-control program (Cuba)	Perez et al. (2011)	Assessed fidelity of intervention, participation of program staff, used semi-structured interviews.	Factors associated with lower fidelity or variable implementation included lack of skills or training, lack of leadership.

Program description (place)	Author (year)	Types of PE used	Usefulness of PE for the program
HIV schools program (South Africa)	Mukoma et al. (2009)	Evaluation in 13 intervention and 13 control schools; assessed factors supporting implementation.	Teacher training, manuals provided, program acceptance, perceived importance of HIV prevention influenced degree of implementation.
Dutch Obesity Intervention in Teenagers (DOiT) weight-gain prevention program for teenagers (Netherlands)	Singh et al. (2009)	PE to assess program reach, implementation, satisfaction and program maintenance.	Low recruitment rate noted; among participating schools, most students reached, program fidelity high.
PE to explain effects of Tai Chi falls-prevention trial	Logghe et al. (2011)	RCT showed no effect on falls-prevention indicators; PE showed low proportion attended, high withdrawal.	PE used as 'explanatory' of a non-effective program.

Process evaluation: used in scaled-up interventions, replication or dissemination studies
(stages 4 and 5 in Figure 2.1)

Health advisers for smoking prevention among disadvantaged women	English et al. (2010)	Multiple methods of PE to assess implementation across settings: ■ how the program fitted into other preventive efforts ■ different adaptations in different contexts.	Identified factors associated with large-scale implementation of a smoking-prevention program using an evidence-based intervention, and continuous training of lay health advisers found useful.
Active for life PE: fidelity and adaptations	Griffin et al. (2010)	Process evaluation of translation of two physical activity programs; high dose delivered and good program fidelity.	Organisations 'adapted' these theory-based programs in different contexts (local 'fit' required).
Process evaluation of: Pool Cool diffusion trial (skin cancer prevention)	Escoffery et al. (2008)	Scaling up of initial efficacy intervention to reduce poolside sun exposure; PE of replication of the intervention in multiple sites.	Implementation was generally good, but was enhanced by having program resources, children enjoying the program, field coordinator support.

Box 4.1 More complex quantitative methods to assess how interventions work

Process evaluation methods can be used by quantitative researchers to understand how programs work; this is through testing theory or theoretical mechanisms directly, using statistical methods to model program data. In particular, researchers test if there are theoretical *mediators*, through which the program exerts its effects. These might be at the individual level (increased confidence to act) or at a community or organsational level. In addition, researchers often report *moderator* analyses, who define whether different subgroups change in different ways following an intervention (Figure 4.1). These methods are methodological (Bauman et al. 2002) but are increasingly reported in the research literature, and describe new quantitative ways of understanding program processes and differential subgroup effectiveness.

The upper panel in Figure 4.1 asks the question whether a tobacco prevention intervention leads directly to a change in smoking status, or whether the intervention changes some intermediary theoretical variable (in this case, self-efficacy—that is, self-confidence—as the 'mediator'), and that increased confidence in turn leads to quitting smoking. The lower panel in the figure shows an example of moderator analysis. A quit-smoking program might result overall in a 20 per cent cessation rate (intervention effects), but researchers are interested in whether program effects are different in subgroups of the population. Here, the effects are explored by gender, and quit rates are greater among women than men. In this example, gender is a moderator (what statisticians call an 'interaction', implying an interaction between gender and the program effect).

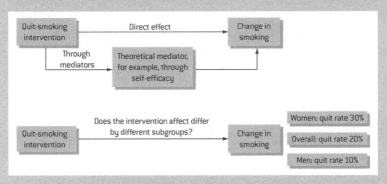

Figure 4.1 Advanced statistical modelling in process evaluation: understanding how interventions work through mediator and moderator analyses

4.3 Summary

Careful, systematic process evaluation provides explanatory information for understanding program effectiveness, as well as providing valuable insights into the practicalities of implementation: what activities occur, under what conditions, by whom and with what level of effort. This knowledge is essential for subsequent replication and dissemination studies. Information from process evaluation is also invaluable in interpreting the impact of evaluation data and their likely causal links to the program. Good process evaluation will ensure that much more is learned and understood about success or failure in achieving defined outcomes. Through this understanding, it is possible to identify the conditions that need to be created to achieve successful outcomes.

By definition, process evaluation should occur throughout the delivery of the program. It can provide a structured account of the elements in a program, assess any variability in program delivery and identify the reasons for such variation. Process evaluation will also assess the reach (that is, the documented participation rate) of the program to its target audience, and the audience's awareness of the program and perceptions of its usefulness and relevance. Finally, process evaluation will describe the strengths and weakness of the program, and explain why and how they worked or did not work.

Process evaluation should be seen as a compulsory part of any health promotion program evaluation. Reflections on the processes of implementation can occur during an intervention, so that corrections and adjustments can be made to improve the likelihood of achieving desired outcomes. In addition, process evaluation data are examined alongside outcome evaluation data at the end of the intervention. Finally, process evaluation is important beyond the individual project or intervention, and can be used in scaled-up programs and replication or dissemination studies as the central evaluation tasks required. This is discussed further in Chapters 6 and 7.

References

Bauman AE, Sallis JF & Dzewaltowski DA et al. 2002, 'Toward a better understanding of the influences on physical activity: the role of determinants, correlates, causal variables, mediators, moderators, and confounders', *American Journal of Preventive Medicine*, vol. 23, no. 2 (supplement), August, pp. 5–14.

Cheadle A, Hsu C & Schwartz PM et al. 2008, 'Involving local health departments in community health partnerships: evaluation results from the partnership for the public's health initiative', *Journal of Urban Health–Bulletin of the New York Academy of Medicine*, vol. 85, no. 2, pp. 162–77.

Colkesen EB, Kraaijenhagen RA & Frings-Dresen MHW et al. 2011, 'Participation in a workplace web-based health risk assessment program', *Occupational Medicine*, vol. 61, no. 8, pp. 586–8.

Collard DCM, Chinapaw MJM & Verhagen E et al. 2010, 'Process evaluation of a school-based physical activity related injury prevention programme using the RE-AIM framework', *BMC Pediatrics*, vol. 10, no. 86.

English KC, Merzel C & Moon-Howard J 2010, 'Translating public health knowledge into practice: development of a lay health advisor perinatal tobacco cessation program', *Journal of Public Health Management and Practice*, vol. 16, no. 3, E9–19.

Eni R & Rowe G 2011, 'Understanding parenting in Manitoba first nations: implications for program development', *Family & Community Health*, vol. 34, no. 3, pp. 221–8.

Escoffery C, Glanz K & Elliott T 2008, 'Process evaluation of the Pool Cool diffusion trial for skin cancer prevention across 2 years', *Health Education Research*, vol. 23, no. 4, pp. 732–43.

Goenka S, Tewari A & Arora M et al. 2010, 'Process evaluation of a tobacco prevention program in Indian schools: methods, results and lessons learnt', *Health Education Research*, vol. 25, no. 6, pp. 917–35.

Griffin SF, Wilcox S & Ory MG et al. 2010, 'Results from the Active for Life process evaluation: program delivery fidelity and adaptations', *Health Education Research*, vol. 25, no. 2, pp. 325–42.

Hargreaves J, Hatcher A & Strange V et al. 2010, 'Process evaluation of the Intervention with Microfinance for AIDS and Gender Equity (IMAGE) in rural South Africa', *Health Education Research*, vol. 25, no. 1, pp. 27–40.

Hong T, Johnson CC & Myers L et al. 2008, 'Process evaluation of an in-school anti-tobacco media campaign in Louisiana', *Public Health Reports*, vol. 123, no. 6, pp. 781–9.

Logghe IHJ, Verhagen AP & Rademaker A et al. 2011, 'Explaining the ineffectiveness of a Tai Chi fall prevention training for community-living older people: a process evaluation alongside a randomized clinical trial (RCT)', *Archives of Gerontology and Geriatrics*, vol. 52, no. 3, pp. 357–62.

Mukoma W, Flisher AJ & Ahmed N et al. 2009, 'Process evaluation of a school-based HIV/AIDS intervention in South Africa', *Scandinavian Journal of Public Health*, vol. 37, pp. 37–47.

Perez D, Lefevre P & Castro M et al. 2011, 'Process-oriented fidelity research assists in evaluation, adjustment and scaling-up of community-based interventions', *Health Policy Plan*, vol. 26, no. 5, pp. 413–22.

Rath S, Nair N & Tripathy PK et al. 2010, 'Explaining the impact of a women's group led community mobilisation intervention on maternal and newborn health outcomes: the Ekjut trial process evaluation', *BMC International Health and Human Rights*, vol. 10, p. 25.

Singh AS, Chinapaw MJM & Brug J et al. 2009, 'Process evaluation of a school-based weight gain prevention program: the Dutch Obesity Intervention in Teenagers (DOiT)', *Health Education Research*, vol. 24, no. 5, pp. 772–7.

5

Evaluation methods for health promotion projects (interventions)

This chapter describes the evaluation processes involved in evidence generation to identify if a discrete program works; this is stage 3 of the stages of evaluation model presented in Chapter 2. The focus of this chapter is to understand research designs used to establish if an intervention works. There is a need for balance between 'scientific' design against public health pragmatism in research design, sample selection and measurement.

Chapters 3 and 4 described the formative and process research methods that support the development of a health promotion project and assessment of whether or not it was implemented as intended. This chapter focuses on the evaluation designs and research methods that are used to test the efficacy and effectiveness of a health promotion intervention. 'Efficacy' implies that the evaluation occurred in ideal circumstances where there was optimal delivery and a high degree of control over the intervention. 'Effectiveness' here means the success of the health promotion project under 'real-world' or 'field' conditions in producing the impact and outcomes that were predicted during the planning of the program as defined in Chapter 1. Did the intervention 'work' and what kind of evidence is provided by the evaluation?

This chapter identifies the evaluation methods used in efficacy and effectiveness studies. These are usually small-scale studies, in selected populations, and are typical of health promotion project evaluations. They use a range of research designs, and can present technical challenges in the recruitment and selection of participants, measurement of outcomes and analysis of results.

Addressing the evaluation challenges for these small-scale or focused projects is the central theme of this chapter. This kind of evaluation work will help to identify 'what works' in health promotion. Chapter 6 addresses issues relating to the evaluation of more complex, multi-component health promotion programs and Chapter 7 deals with research issues around the evaluation of replication and dissemination studies.

This chapter starts with a discussion of research methods and evaluation designs required for discrete projects (projects usually using a single intervention strategy), for example, a social media intervention to encourage healthy eating; a school curriculum to teach young people about HIV risk; or a social cognitive theory–led behaviour change intervention to support regular smokers to quit. Each of these health promotion projects delivers a well-delineated 'intervention' to a well-defined population.

5.1   Evaluation designs for health promotion projects

The term 'evaluation design' describes the set of tasks to systematically examine the effects of a health promotion intervention. The purpose of a good evaluation design is to create confidence that the health promotion intervention caused any changes that were observed. To achieve this, we need to ensure that:

- the program was optimally *developed and planned* (formative evaluation), *implemented* as intended, and *reached* the target audience (process evaluation);
- the processes of *recruitment of people* into the intervention are described, for example, who they were and how they were selected;
- the best possible *measurements* were used to assess the impact and outcomes from the intervention (the results);
- the best possible *research design* was used to assess the effects of the intervention;
- no *alternative explanations* exist for the results, so that we can be confident that the results observed are attributable to the intervention;
- we can *identify* the individuals, population groups or subgroups to whom these observed intervention effects do and do not apply;
- we can *identify* how and why the program worked (or did not work) for the whole, or for subsets of, the target group.

Put simply, the better the evaluation design and methods that we use in assessing impact and outcome, the more confident we can be that the intervention caused the observed effects of a program and that these did not occur by chance, or due to other factors or influences. As indicated in Chapter 4, the first step in any evaluation should be systematic process evaluation, to identify whether or not the program was implemented as planned, and 'delivered' to the whole group or sample intended to benefit from the intervention. This chapter identifies the elements of good impact evaluation methodology, starting with characteristics of people who participate in the intervention; the choice of research designs; methods of program measurement; and the search for alternative explanations for observed program effects.

The research process in an evidence-generating intervention

Figure 5.1 shows the key features of this chapter, from initial recruitment of participants to process and impact evaluation and to replication and dissemination (the latter are discussed in Chapter 7). The first step is to identify the group of people who might enrol in the intervention.

Identification of the target group

This is the potential target group among which to seek participants for the intervention. The identification of the target group, and its size and composition, may also influence the types of evaluation methods used. For example, with a very large national program, the evaluation design will be different to that for a small, focused community. Further, the measurements possible will also be influenced by the characteristics of the target population, and their *health literacy*.

It is important to identify who participates in public health programs, and whether they are typical (or *representative*) of the whole population. Before or during this phase, formative evaluation is conducted to establish best practice in this kind of intervention. Once the intervention begins, people are defined as 'included' in intervention or program, and from that point onwards, process and impact evaluation are carried out. After the intervention has concluded, follow-up assessment may be useful to establish if any changes were maintained. The concept of participation is important to understanding

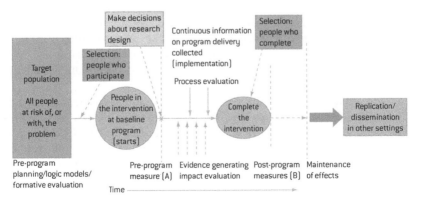

Figure 5.1 The evaluation process

the potential for the results of the program to be *generalised* to other settings. The starting point is identifying people in the target population who are potentially eligible for an intervention. For example, a smoking-prevention intervention might target all pregnant women who smoke, but only 10 per cent of at-risk women might actually enrol in the program and of these, only half might complete the intervention (see Figure 5.1).

It is important to assess the differences between participants who are eligible from those who actually enrol at the start of the program, and those who complete the program.

The importance of selecting a representative sample of subjects in a study and the risks of selection bias are discussed further in the next section.

Choice of evaluation (or research) designs

The next part of the research process is the choice of an evaluation design (also known as a *research design* or *study design*). The evaluation design should be the 'best possible' in the context of the program, its implementation and in meeting the expectations of the different stakeholders. For example, a program to increase the use of injury-prevention strategies in the workplace may have a different 'best possible' research design when compared to a community-based program to prevent falls and injuries in a group of home-bound older people. The research design is implemented from the point labelled 'X' on Figure 5.2 on page 74.

Controlled trials

There is a hierarchy of research designs from the 'most scientific', which use *experimental* designs and are commonly referred to as **randomised controlled trials (RCTs)**. This is illustrated in design 1, shown in Figure 5.2. The people who receive the intervention are not predetermined, with individuals randomly allocated to receive or not receive the program. Every individual or group has an equal chance of being offered or not offered the program. This *random allocation* of individuals makes it more likely that differences (such as personal background or existing health status) between a population receiving an intervention and a population not receiving an intervention can be minimised. It also reduces the possibility that observed changes in the intervention group are due to 'chance' effects caused by existing differences in the two populations, and raises the likelihood that the intervention caused any such changes.

Once the individuals have been randomly allocated to the *intervention or comparison (control) groups*, a baseline assessment is made of their characteristics (such as age, gender and the objects of the intervention, for example, smoking behaviour or healthy eating patterns) to determine that the intervention and *control* groups are comparable (shown as 'A' in Figure 5.1). Measurements are then performed on the same individuals after the intervention has been completed to assess change in the objects of the intervention, and to test that change for *statistical significance* (shown as 'B' in Figure 5.1). The quality of an experimental evaluation design can be examined according to well-established criteria, such as the comprehensive 25-item CONSORT checklist (Consolidated Standards of Reporting of Trials). Some of these items are summarised in Appendix 1.

In addition to individual-level randomisation (examples 1 and 2 in Table 5.1 on page 72), it is possible to randomise at the level of communities or groups, for example, randomising whole populations in workplaces, primary care centres or schools to receive an intervention; this is known as a cluster RCT (Figure 5.2, and examples 3 and 4 in Table 5.1). For example, within the same school, students are likely to share common influences on their health behaviour or beliefs, which means we need to take account statistically of this clustering. These common influences on students' behaviours and beliefs make it appropriate to consider them as a 'group' in a research study. This type of research design is well-suited to interventions that are intended to be delivered to whole groups (such as a school class), or interventions based on a modification to the environment that might have an impact on a whole group (for example, the introduction of healthy food options in a work site's canteen).

A third RCT design is the stepped-wedge design, where units or groups are allocated sequentially to an intervention, so that waiting-list groups can be compared as the intervention rolls out across a population (Figure 5.2, and example 5 in Table 5.1). This is useful across a large region, where for financial or other practical reasons an implementation needs to be rolled out over time.

Because randomised trials usually involve some individuals receiving an intervention and some not, it is important to make sure that randomised trials are ethical, and that nobody fails to receive the care that they need. In these circumstances 'usual care' or minimal interventions are often provided. For example, in a clinic or primary care setting, it may be possible to randomly allocate groups of patients with diabetes to receive a comprehensive education and skills development program, and others to be allocated to a control group consisting of their 'usual clinic care'. In such circumstances it is important to follow ethical protocols, and ensure that your evaluation study has received approval from an appropriate institutional ethics review board.

It is also important to keep the people in intervention and control groups separated from each other as much as is practically possible. One of the challenges faced by evaluators is to ensure that there is no **contamination** of the control group. For example, sometimes those receiving an intervention can share information or program resources with control group participants, who are not intended to receive the intervention. This increases the chances that this non-intervention (control) group will make changes that are the object of the intervention, and such *contamination* makes it (statistically) more difficult to detect the effects of a program. This is particularly challenging in health promotion interventions that are designed to reach whole populations— hence the use of cluster RCTs, randomising by whole settings or geographically discrete units, as a research design alternative.

Although the use of experimental designs is always preferable, for the reasons indicated above it is often impractical to evaluate a health promotion program using an RCT design. This kind of design may require substantial funding and good control over the intervention delivery. It is most necessary when there is a high need for 'generating evidence' of intervention efficacy. This might be when a program is being tested for the first time, or is expensive (and would be costly to reproduce widely), or may be controversial, or is considered risky.

Given the diversity of settings and complexity of interventions, alternative designs may be considered. These provide less rigorous evidence of program effectiveness, but may be the most feasible in many situations. 'Best practice' in health promotion evaluation will always require consideration of the 'optimal against the possible' in evaluation design. These non-RCT designs are categorised as 'quasi-experimental' and 'pre-experimental' designs.

Quasi-experimental and pre-experimental designs

Quasi-experimental designs have a clearly defined *control* or *comparison* population: a population who do not receive an intervention, and against which intervention group effects could be compared (designs 4, 4a and 4b in Figure 5.2, and examples 5–8 in Table 5.1). Here, the group receiving the intervention is predetermined and is not randomly assigned, so there is a greater chance that any observed changes may be influenced by differences between intervention and control groups or communities, and not caused by the intervention. This is especially the case when the intervention is delivered to enthusiastic volunteers who are then compared with a less committed 'control' population.

As is the case with RCTs, the quality of the results from quasi-experimental studies is dependent on the size and representativeness of the study population, the use of valid and reliable measures before and after the intervention, the implementation of the intervention as planned, and optimal approaches to analysis and interpretation. The analyses may need to be statistically adjusted for baseline differences between intervention and control groups or communities (for example, differences in the age, gender or social background of participants).

RCTs have the same individuals assessed before and after the program. Quasi-experimental studies may also involve the same people (**cohort**) followed up from pre- to post-program, but some population interventions are evaluated using different (independent) *cross-section* samples of people from the target population to assess changes over time. This is referred to as a *repeat* **cross-sectional study**, and while feasible in many health promotion program evaluations, it is not as methodologically strong as a cohort study for explaining how and why observed changes occurred.

Quasi-experimental designs may be a practical and pragmatic approach to evaluating many health promotion interventions. This is especially the case where interventions are directed at whole populations or large regions (where the allocation of individuals to intervention and non-intervention groups is impossible). Examples include a region-wide immunisation program, a national mass media campaign or large-scale preventive service offered over a large region. In these examples, careful quasi-experimental designs are feasible design for assessing the effectiveness of these programs. Examples of interventions using a quasi-experimental design are shown in Table 5.1 on pages 72–3.

Another type of quasi-experimental evaluation design is a **time-series design**. In this evaluation design there are multiple pre-intervention measurements, followed by the health promotion intervention, and then several post-intervention measurements (design types 5 and 5a in Figure 5.2 on page 74). Here, trends in the measure of interest can be observed (for example, smoking prevalence, or preventive screening rates, or access to a health promotion service), and the intervention effect can be judged by changes to the outcomes of interest over time and whether the intervention group showed significantly greater change than the comparison group. Time-series designs may be useful in the evaluation of policy interventions, as they allow for structured observation of change in a population where a policy has been introduced with little consideration for the evaluation of its effects (for example, a ban on smoking in specific places). An example is shown in Table 5.1, using repeated population surveys to evaluate alcohol policy and marketing.

The time-series design approach is strengthened by the addition of one or more comparison groups or regions, which also have trend data (design type 5a in Figure 5.2). This is a quasi-experimental design as the population receiving the intervention determined by the program planners (and is not randomly assigned), so there is a risk that any observed changes may have been influenced by factors or events other than the intervention. This type of quasi-experimental design is particularly useful where there are routine data collections by health authorities or other agencies (such as pap smear tests for cervical cancer screening) and, for example, a mass media campaign encouraging screening in one region can be compared with a region not specifically encouraging screening, with the outcome being a change in screening rates over time.

The last group of designs have been described as *pre-experimental*. These provide the weakest evidence and should only be used after other possibilities have been considered. A 'before–after' one group evaluation design (**pre-post study**; type 6 in Figure 5.2) is a relatively weak design as it does not provide compelling evidence that the health promotion intervention *caused* any observed changes; as indicated previously, people change their behaviours for many reasons, and not only in response to structured interventions. Nonetheless, this simple evaluation design does give some estimate of change, and is often used in pilot studies to estimate the likely effect of an intervention.

However, in some circumstances, a 'before–after' single group design is the only design possible in health promotion or public health. An example would be the evaluation of a large-scale national campaign. Here, it may not be possible to have a comparison population or region, if the national campaign targets the entire population. This type of study design is strengthened by having multiple baseline pre-intervention measures (design type 5a in Figure 5.2), and ideally multiple post-intervention measures to assess the maintenance of program effects.

The weakest design is the one-group 'post-program only' evaluation (example 9 in Table 5.1). This is where people are only surveyed or assessed following the program. This design should never be used for assessing program effects as it is not possible to claim that reported changes (for example, in health behaviours) were caused by the intervention. Such a design may be useful for collecting process evaluation measures, such as participants' assessment of their use of program components, but should never be considered for assessing program impact. In addition, qualitative evaluation methods (example 10 in Table 5.1), such as case series approaches or focus group discussions, could also be classified as 'pre-experimental'. However, such qualitative evaluations may generate process evaluation information and contribute to understanding the program, even if these methods do not generate 'causal' evidence of program effectiveness.

In summary, the first stage is deciding on the best possible evaluation design to meet circumstances, but is not enough to guarantee a successful evaluation. Several important technical issues must also be addressed to ensure the quality of evidence provided. These include participation rates of those eligible for the program (see Table 5.2), the measurements chosen, and the analytical methods used to interpret the data. Each of these is considered in the remainder of this chapter.

Table 5.1 Examples of research design

Randomised trial designs (experimental studies)		
Example 1: individual-level randomised controlled trial (RCT)	Fledderus et al. (2010) examined the efficacy of an intervention to reduce psychosocial distress among 93 adults. The intervention aimed to promote positive mental health.	Individuals were randomised to intervention and control groups, and the intervention group scored better on validated measures of 'wellbeing' than the controls, at three-month follow-up.
Example 2: individual-level RCT	Wing et al. (2010) described an intensive lifestyle intervention for 5145 adults with type 2 diabetes, the LOOK AHEAD trial, and its impact on cardiovascular risk factors.	Individuals were randomised to the LOOK AHEAD intensive intervention, or the diabetes support and education control group. This efficacy trial showed significantly greater improvements at 12 months in weight, fitness, blood pressure and cholesterol levels, compared to controls.
Example 3: cluster randomised trial	Caria et al. (2011) aimed to assess the efficacy of a new school-based substance-use curriculum, around promoting social influences, in 143 schools in seven European countries.	Used cluster RCT, randomised schools to intervention or control schools. Results showed intervention curriculum effectively delayed problem alcohol use.
Example 4: cluster randomised trial	MANAS trial (Patel et al. 2010) in 24 regions of Goa, India, testing an intervention where health counsellors target anxiety and depression among adults. Counselling was supplemented by referral and clinical treatment through primary care settings.	Regions were randomly allocated to receive the intervention or be control communities. People with mental health problems in the intervention regions were more likely to have recovered from their mental health problems than control residents.
Example 5: stepped-wedge design	Killam et al. (2010) described an intervention to implement antiretroviral treatment for HIV-infected women through antenatal clinics, where the implementation happened over two months across clinics in Lusaka, Zambia. (It is not clear if implementation was done according to a random schedule or simply by convenience.)	This stepped-wedge design implemented the treatment over time across clinics and assessed how well the intervention worked; results demonstrated a two-fold increase in treatment initiation and in early start to treatment in the clinics where the therapy was introduced.

Quasi-experimental evaluation studies		
Example 6: quasi-experimental design	Shelley et al. (2008) examined the effects of policy interventions compared to policy-community approaches to tobacco control among Chinese Americans.	Quasi-experiment with surveys of target population (before and after) in intervention and control regions.
Example 7: time-series design	Dumsha et al. (2011) explored whether the introduction of sweetened flavoured alcohol-containing drinks (alcopops) resulted in increases in alcohol consumption by American teenagers.	Using multiple repeated adolescent health survey data, in a time-series design, it was shown that increases did occur in several population subgroups after the alcohol beverage industry had introduced 'alcopops'.
Example 8: pre–post single group design	Vadheim et al. (2010) reported on a translational study (replication of an evidence-based study: see Chapter 7), testing if a known effective diabetes prevention program can be replicated in rural Montana (USA).	Pre–post design of 101 people at risk of diabetes (uncontrolled study)—showed effects similar to those in the previous efficacy trials on weight loss and increased physical activity.
Example 9: post-only design	McConnell et al. (2012) evaluated the 'Triple P positive parenting program' among 923 parents and their children.	Post-only surveys showed parents receiving greater amounts of the program were more satisfied, but no different on stress, child interactions or problem behaviours. Functionally this is no different to process evaluation, and no inference can be made on outcomes (parental stress, child problem behaviours).
Example 10: qualitative designs only used in program evaluation	Louis-Nance et al. (2012) aimed to identify the effects of an education program about human papilloma virus for mothers and daughters.	Qualitative methods only, focus groups and interviews with mothers and daughters. Identified common themes, specific areas that improved, and areas that increased mother–daughter communication. Only qualitative methods, no statistical testing.

Experimental research designs

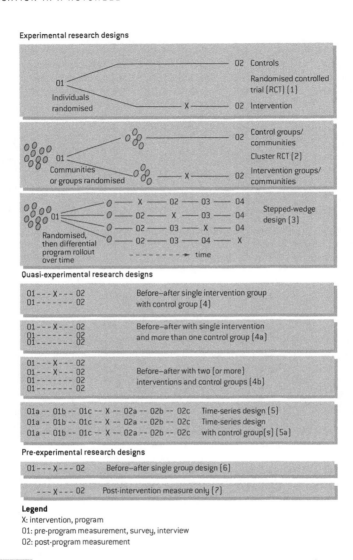

Legend

X: intervention, program
01: pre-program measurement, survey, interview
02: post-program measurement

Figure 5.2 Quantitative evaluation designs for individual programs (stage 3 of Figure 2.1), ranked from 'most scientific' experimental designs to less scientific 'pre-experimental' designs

5.2 Selection bias and sampling

The issues surrounding selection effects have been mentioned earlier, in the way in which people from the target population end up in the 'evaluation' study and whether they are *representative* of the target population. Methods for minimising *selection bias* are shown in Box 5.1.

Sampling and recruitment

In small-scale interventions, we can include everyone who is targeted for intervention in the evaluation. When planning large community-wide programs (that reach thousands of people) this is not practical for the purposes of evaluation. In such circumstances, we sample a subset of individuals from the population to assess the impact of the program. By using *random sampling*, the effects of the program on a **random sample** can be considered applicable (generalisable) to the whole source population.

Random sampling implies that a list of the target population exists, and that people can be selected for the study at random. Examples of such population-level lists include census data, health clinic or health insurance lists, employee payroll lists, lists of populations of patients registered in primary care, school lists of enrolled pupils, and even telephone directories (in locations where there are still high numbers of fixed-line telephones). A random sample can be drawn systematically (such as every tenth person), or using a computer to generate

Box 5.1 Minimising selection bias

The evidence generated by a study is more persuasive if you can demonstrate that the population you have studied is 'typical' of (*generalisable to*) the general population. By achieving this, you make it more likely that the effects that you have observed are applicable to a broader population.

In developing a study design, it is important to minimise any sources of *bias* that may affect the results. Bias is where something differs systematically from the true situation, or contributes to conclusions that differ from the 'true situation'. Biases may come from a range of sources including the *selection* of participants (enrolment and recruitment of participants in a study/intervention, and their retention for the duration of the study). Bias can also come from systematic *measurement* errors.

Selection biases include differences between those, from the target population, who enrol in an intervention and those who do not participate (known as **non-response bias**); in addition, selection effects may be noted during an intervention, comparing those who **drop out** or do not complete the intervention with those who complete it. Participants may have different social, educational or other attributes, or have greater interest and motivation to change that distinguish them from those not enrolled or not those who do not complete the intervention.

To obtain generalisable evidence, it is important to try to obtain a representative sample for any study and, in intervention studies, to maintain a high participation rate. Maintaining people in evaluation studies may be facilitated by not requiring too much in terms of assessment, by active support and encouragement, and sometimes by the provision of incentives for continued participation.

a list of 10 numbers chosen at random from 100 possible numbers. Then, the 10 chosen people (or work sites or settings) will be included in the *sample*.

In cases where no population 'list' or record exists, it will not be possible or practical to achieve a true random sample from a population, for example, among homeless people or other highly marginalised groups. Other examples of ways in which sampling occurs are shown in Table 5.2. These include *convenient samples* of volunteers and *snowball sampling*.

Table 5.2 Sampling methods used in the evaluation of health promotion interventions

	Recruitment of participants to a small health promotion trial *[for example, a trial of an education program to increase self-management skills in people with asthma or heart disease]*	Sampling of people to evaluate a large-scale intervention *[for example, a community education program to increase the rate of mammography screening for all women aged 40–59]*
Optimal sampling method ↑ ↓ Least generisable sampling method	■ Random sampling from the population of people with asthma or with heart disease. ■ Sampling from a defined database of people. ■ Sampling from numerous community groups and clinic settings—even if non-random, may show enough diversity to be generalisable. ■ 'Snowball samples', where hard-to-reach individuals can be found and sampled through social networks. ■ Volunteers with asthma or heart disease recruited through newspaper advertisements, or through local hospital clinics.	■ Random sampling of all women aged 40–59 is measured (sampled from the whole at-risk population). ■ Other variants of random sampling: – random sampling with increased samples (oversampling) of specific groups of interest—such as an ethnic group that is less likely to be screened; – universal sampling (if the population is small, it is possible to survey everybody). ■ Non-random (convenient) sampling, for example: – street intercept samples; – samples of middle-aged women from a particular cultural grouping; – other convenience samples from women attending a group or club or belonging to an organisation.

Sampling techniques are used to ensure that the population that is studied is representative of the whole population intended to benefit from an intervention, and *statistical tests* can be used to assess the importance (referred to as *significance*) of the observed changes between the intervention and comparison samples. In general, the larger the study sample is, the greater the chance of showing a statistically significant difference between the intervention and comparison groups.

5.3 Statistical significance and data analysis

A serious examination of biostatistics is beyond the scope of this book, but an understanding of some basic statistical concepts is needed during the planning phase of a program, and for the critical appraisal and interpretation of evaluation findings. Further reading is recommended at the end of this chapter. The purpose of statistical methods is to help us interpret the quantitative evaluation data produced from an evaluation study. No matter how good the quality of the data collected, if it is not analysed and interpreted well, it will not produce useful information on the success or otherwise of an intervention.

Sample size calculations

Initial statistical considerations occur before the program starts. We need to know how many people we need to include in a study to be confident that the results we get are likely to be true (**sample size**). For example, an obesity prevention program might determine that an objective for the intervention group is to lose an average of three kilograms over 12 months. In this case, the proposed objective to lose an average of three kilograms over 12 months has been made on the basis of previous studies that have shown this to be feasible and likely to produce health benefits. It is an estimate of the proposed **effect size** that the intervention is trying to achieve, and in a defined time period.

With known measures (and with an understanding of their variation) it is possible to calculate the number of people that will be needed in a study population to detect an effect of a pre-specified size. Obviously, this sample size calculation should be done before the evaluation starts, as it will guide program recruitment.

Statistical methods and statistical testing

Statistical methods are used to determine whether the results observed might have occurred by chance. This is referred to as the level of *statistical significance*. Statistical significance describes the probability of the observed results (i.e. the difference in a target outcome when comparing the measure before and after an intervention, and/or between intervention and control groups) occurring by chance. Statistical significance is often described in terms of probability of the observed finding occurring by chance; these statements of probability are described as *p values*, which are often shown in published papers as p<0.05 or p<0.01). This simply means that there is a one-in-20 or one-in-100 probability of an observed outcome occurring by chance respectively. A related statistical concept is the use of **confidence intervals** around an observed outcome. In this case confidence intervals describe how likely are the true results in the underlying population to be outside the range described by the confidence limits.

Statistical tests require consideration of the type and distribution of the data collected, specifically whether data are *continuous* measures or *categorical*. A continuous measure can take many values, and can be described in terms of an average (mean) value and its variation (standard deviation). For example, blood pressure, or the number of cigarettes smoked each day, or weight in kilograms can be continuous measurements. Some outcomes are just described as a category (for example, 'improved/did not improve'; 'smoker/non-smoker'). Different statistical tests are required for continuous data (these include *parametric tests*, such as t-tests, linear regression models and so on), compared to analytical approaches to data in categories, which require the use of chi-squared statistics, and relative risks or odds ratios. These are illustrated by examples of 'continuous data' and 'categorical data' in data from a hypothetical intervention in Appendix 2.

Other factors influencing interpretation of results

In analysing results from an evaluation, consideration has to be given to whether the results observed might be due to some other factors, either in the data or external to the program. Internal factors might contribute in subtle ways—it may be that one group improves most because it is more socially connected or has greater confidence about achieving the outcomes. External factors might contribute to observed changes in outcomes in both intervention and control groups. For example, unpredicted media interest in an issue in the middle of an intervention could impact on public response to that intervention (positively or negatively). In addition, other background factors that need to be considered include national or global trends; for example, in some countries, tobacco use has declined and community views on restricting smoking in indoor environments have strengthened over a prolonged period. A health promotion program in a defined community to address these issues would have to consider the rate of background changes in public attitudes and behaviours, and assess whether the program could produce effects greater than these existing **secular trends**.

Similarly, the background effects of large-scale national programs may reduce or confuse the effect of a local-level intervention. For example, the impact of a national media campaign to promote uptake of immunisation against influenza among older people might completely mask the impact of a local project conducted to improve immunisation uptake by patients in an individual health clinic.

Finally, there may be extraneous factors associated with the intervention and with the outcomes of interest that may distort the estimates of program effectiveness. These are known as **confounding factors** and should be considered in analysis. As they are somewhat technical, they are beyond the scope of this volume (see Bauman 2002).

It is worth noting that it may not always be 'positive change' that indicates program success. For example, given the increases in obesity in many countries, a local program that demonstrated no change in obesity prevalence over five years at the same time as national prevalence was rising would be a relative success. In such circumstances, having a control region or prior serial national monitoring data is useful, and allows this intervention to be appraised as a successful innovation in preventing the expected weight gain.

5.4 Health promotion measurement

A fundamental component of the evaluation of a health promotion intervention is the accurate and consistent measurement of impact and outcomes. Measurement is the assessment of phenomena, and can use either qualitative or quantitative methods or both. Understanding the characteristics of good quality measures is important in improving the credibility of evaluation findings. We assess changes in specific measures to determine the impact and effectiveness of health promotion projects by detecting changes in health promotion outcome such as changes in (measures of) knowledge and community attitudes; and intermediate health outcome measures, such as changes in health behaviours or environments.

This section describes some of the challenges in measurement in project evaluation. Many measurements are based on self-reported information (collected by questionnaires completed online or on paper, or by telephone or face-to-face interview). Other measures are objective, directly observable assessments of phenomena (for example, body weight, blood pressure or immunisation status). Measurement may be of individual attributes (knowledge, attitudes, social norms) or may assess characteristics of organisations, environments, communities or systems.

The definition and measurement of *intermediate health outcomes*, such as health behaviours and healthy environments, and the *health promotion outcomes* that may influence them, have taxed the skills of researchers for decades. Measurement development has focused on assessment of individual behaviours, such as smoking or alcohol use, rather than measures of health promotion processes. The latter, for example, measures of social mobilisation or health literacy, are less well-developed.

One important issue is the difference between **measures and indicators**. The latter are often proxy or indirect measures that reflect a generally related area, and can be used at a large scale to monitor processes or progress. Evaluation work uses indicators to assess health promotion outcomes and typically uses reliable and valid measures for intermediate and outcome assessment. An example of the difference can be seen if we think about measures of, first, adolescent health, and second, social capital. For adolescents, measures might be rates of binge drinking of alcohol, illicit drug use or individual-level mental health measures; at the community level, process indicators might include education system provision, access to youth facilities, or criminal conviction rates for drug possession. Both indicators and measures could be included in an evaluation of adolescent substance use prevention in a defined community. Similarly, in a study to improve social capital, we might use individual-level quantitative measures, such as sense of coherence, trust and social support. In addition, we may also use community-level indicators such as poverty, crime rates and safety. In many projects, the indicators are routinely collected, and may corroborate trends in phenomena of interest to decision-makers.

Measurement reliability and validity

We need to be sure that what we measure accurately reflects the purpose of the intervention and can be sensibly used as the basis for an evaluation of the intervention. Key elements of any measurements are that they are reliable and valid. Poor measurement is one source of bias that may lead to erroneous conclusions about program effects. The concept of 'measurement bias' is shown in Box 5.2.

Box 5.2 Measurement error and measurement bias

Measures are not perfect: there is some error in all measurement, compared to the 'true state' that is being assessed. One kind of measurement error is 'random variation', as some attributes vary naturally when measured at different times. An example of this is blood sugar, which might be higher if measured soon after a meal.

Another problem with measurement is 'bias', which is the amount that the observed measurement differs from the 'true' measurement. Sometimes we measure the 'true value' or close to it, as our only measurement; for example, cholesterol levels or immunisation status are assessed using objective measures. In other circumstances, we can ask people to report their smoking status or weight, and we can assess how much this differs compared to an objective measure of these phenomena. Although we can assess how variable self-report measurements are—that is, we can estimate random variation—it may be more difficult to know how far they differ from the 'truth'.

In some cases, we can compare self-reports, of smoking status or weight, against some 'true' measure or 'criterion measurement'. It is more difficult to assess the measurement bias in more subjective self-report measures, for example, of 'attitudes' or 'social capital', and here we may need special techniques adapted from the social sciences (psychometric techniques) to assess measurement validity.

Poor quality measurements can produce either **type 1** or **type 2 errors**. For example, if there is a poor quality measurement in our evaluation (one with too much random variability or one with too much bias or invalid measurement) then error in measurement may preclude our finding a significant difference following an intervention. An example of this could be the measurement of weight—self-report may be biased, and poor scales may show too much variation. Therefore, using good, reproducible measures that are not biased is an important step in interpreting evaluation findings.

Test–re-test reliability refers to the stability of a measure, assessing the extent to which, each time the measure is used, it will measure the same thing. The most common method used to test reliability is the repeat administration of the measurement on the same people, using the same administration procedures, within a short period of time. For example, if the same person answers a set of questions on self-confidence in the same way within a relatively short period of time (1–2 weeks), the measurement can be considered stable and reliable.

Testing for reliability is important even when the object of study can be observed directly, for example, when observing and rating the characteristics of an environment (such as a house or a school). In this case, reliability can be determined by the level of agreement between two observers or 'raters' of the same phenomenon. This is known as *inter-rater reliability*. If there is inter-rater disagreement, then strict guidelines need to be developed to standardise data collection.

Validity is the assessment of the 'truth' of a measurement. A question, scale or test is considered *valid* to the extent that it measures what it intended to measure. A reliable measurement is not necessarily a valid measurement, since you may measure the wrong thing, but do so consistently.

Validity can be assessed objectively. For example, it is possible to measure objectively cotinine in a saliva or blood sample to detect recent tobacco use. This would be an excellent biochemical test of the validity of self-reported questions on smoking behaviour. Although desirable, such objective measures are not always available, practical or affordable.

Measurement of attitudes and beliefs, and self-efficacy do not lend themselves to such objective verification, and other types of measurement validation techniques are needed, usually using methods developed in the social sciences. These include whether the items are considered relevant by experts (referred to as **face validity**), and cover all dimensions of interest (referred to as **content validity**). It is challenging to develop valid measures of concepts such as 'social capital' or 'capacity-building' where experts do not agree on the constituent elements of the concept. This depends on an understanding of the relationship between *concepts, variables* and *constructs*. A **concept** is a theoretical idea used to describe a phenomenon that is not directly observable. Concepts have to be turned into measureable *variables*, which are validly and reliably assessed and show variation among people. Variables may be single questions or *items*, or summarised as composite **scales or scores**. How well the items or questions 'fit' into the score or scale can be assessed by estimating the **internal consistency** of the items. The process of turning items into scores uses psychometric statistical techniques, which describe the measurement properties of these underlying constructs and how well the items are related to the construct. This is called **construct validity**.

The examples provided in Appendix 3 help understand these different types of reliability and validity. The purpose here is for readers to become familiar with the terms used to describe measurement properties, and to understand the context and purposes for which the test is used. This is necessary because many published papers use these terms, and an understanding of these terms helps with critical appraisal of the quality of measurements used. Further reading, or consultation with a statistical measurement expert, is recommended before using them in a program evaluation.

The uses of measurement in evaluation

The purpose of a health promotion intervention is to produce change in a range of determinants of health and thereby improve health. To this end, a measure should be capable of changing in response to an intervention. This is known as measurement **responsiveness** or *sensitivity to change*. All types of measures that you might use need to be of known responsiveness—that is, they can demonstrate change. This is true of measures of a discrete behaviour, such as breastfeeding or smoking, but is also true of more subjective program outcomes, for example, a program that is trying to change measures of public opinion about restricting smoking inside buildings; this measure needs to be shown to be both reliable (stable), and yet sufficiently sensitive to change in response to an intervention targeting community values in the environments in which smoking might occur.

A hypothetical time-series design in a program evaluation is shown in Figure 5.3, with monthly measurements. The figure shows the mean outcome score for two different measures of 'self-confidence' that might have been used in an intervention to improve confidence among young people. This figure shows both measurement *reliability* and *responsiveness*. Mean scores are shown on the y-axis, and time in months on the x-axis. Measure 1 (solid line) is stable (*reliable*) during serial administrations over the months May to September, with the mean scores being similar, around a value of 13–14. This shows that the measure does not change in the absence of an intervention. When the intervention occurs in October, the self-confidence score shows *responsiveness*, increasing to a value of 21 immediately after the intervention.

By contrast, Measure 2 (dotted line) has poor measurement properties for two reasons. It shows great variability pre-intervention, showing substantial fluctuation (is not *reliable*), and then fails to show any *responsiveness* to the

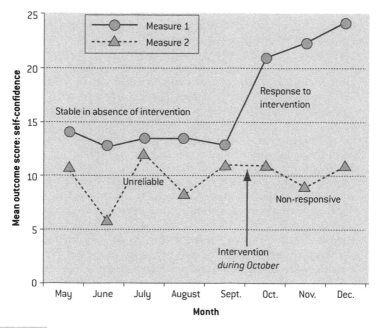

Figure 5.3 Reliability (reproducibility) and responsiveness of measurement

intervention. Hence, this measure will show possible effects in the absence of an intervention due to random measurement fluctuations, and will fail to show an effect when exposed to the October intervention (both *type 1 and type 2* errors), and hence, its use will lead to the wrong conclusion about the program's effects.

It is almost impossible to remove all sources of error and bias from the different measurements that are used in a health promotion evaluation. Other measurement problems and ways of addressing them are shown in Box 5.3. It is important that a researcher minimises their effect on a study and acknowledges the potential for error and bias in discussing the results of a

Box 5.3 Other measurement issues that can influence evaluation results

These include:

- *Response bias as a consequence of simply being observed*—for example, people may report 'socially desirable' answers to sensitive issues, such as substance use, sexual behaviours or domestic violence. Even the mode of administration of a questionnaire, for example, by interview compared to anonymous questionnaire, can influence the measurements obtained. These biases can be reduced by using questions presented in a neutral form, and by offering anonymity or confidentiality where possible.

- *Response bias as a consequence of sensitisation to the issue*—for example, where a person is asked the same questions on repeat occasions. This is particularly a risk in control populations where repeatedly asking someone about their attitudes or behaviours might influence participants to take action that they might not otherwise have taken. If a person who smokes is asked in some detail about their smoking habit on repeated occasions, this in itself might prompt him or her to attempt to quit. This bias can be minimised by undertaking *cross-sectional* surveys of different subjects before and after an intervention, rather than conducting surveys with the same *cohort*.

- *Response changes as a consequence of the maturation of a group or cohort*—for example, at the extremes of age. Longitudinal studies of adolescents may show changes in attitudes or beliefs as a consequence of growing up, such as changes in experience and physical maturation, which may be due to maturation processes, not an intervention. Similarly, older adults may show declines in measures of cognitive abilities or functional status as a consequence of ageing, which may attenuate any positive intervention effect. These changes are not necessarily a source of bias, but need to be considered in the analysis of change over time in a cohort. In the same way, changes to the composition of communities over time may mean that serial cross-sectional survey samples from the same geographical area differ in socio-demographic attributes; if serial surveys are used to evaluate programs, then efforts to account for these differences are required.

study. It is also important for practitioners to be aware of potential error and bias when critically assessing the quality of evidence provided by any health promotion program evaluation discussed in a report or peer-reviewed journal.

Measurement across different stages of evaluation

Each stage in the planning and evaluation process may require different measures and pose different measurement challenges. For example, in program planning and design, routinely collected information on mortality, morbidity and health behaviours might be used to prioritise health problems for intervention. In assessing program implementation, process evaluation measures of participation and of program quality can be used. These measures are not generally routinely available and may need to be specially designed for the project, or at least adapted for use from another project evaluation. Assessment of the short-term impact of a project will often depend on measures of health promotion outcomes, changes in knowledge, self-efficacy or social attitudes; and, over time, changes in behaviour or in the environment can be measured. Longer term health outcome measurement may be possible through the use of epidemiological data on mortality and morbidity. Beyond assessment of the effectiveness of a program (stage 4 evaluation), evaluation of the quality of dissemination requires measures of spread or diffusion of the programs into communities (see Chapter 6). Examples of measures at different stages of evaluation are shown in Table 5.3.

Table 5.3 Measurement at different stages of program evaluation

Stage of program and measurement needs	Examples of measures	Measurement challenges and pitfalls
Program planning and design—formative evaluation	Measures that assess responses of the target group to testing of program materials; perception of stakeholders of program's likely success.	Sufficient sample size and sample variation to assess the generalisability of formative or pilot evaluation findings.
Program implementation; process measures; implementation indicators	Number or proportion of people attending program; number or percentage of professionals participating; program delivered as intended; measures of environmental changes carried out as planned; measures of interagency partnerships developed as planned.	Reliability and validity of process measures; known measurement properties of indicators such as audits of program attendance, satisfaction measures, measures of community partnership and engagement.

(continued)

Table 5.3 *continued*

Stage of program and measurement needs	Examples of measures	Measurement challenges and pitfalls
Health promotion outcomes; individual level	Awareness of health issues; cognitive changes such as self-efficacy, intention to be more active, beliefs.	Psychometric properties, test–re-test repeatability and construct validation of cognitive measures, social support and social capital measures.
Supra-individual measures	Social supports; enhanced social influences; social environment; social capital (collective efficacy).	Reliable and valid measures needed
Intermediate health outcomes (impact)	Behavioural changes; definition of general behaviours; whether there are specific domains of measurement.	Measurement properties including criterion validity, for example, of self-report diet or physical activity; whether measurement domains are part of same construct; assessment and testing of *mediator* (and *moderator*) variables.
Physical environmental measures	Changes made to physical environments completed.	Validity of environmental measures; inter-rater agreement using audit tools.
Community-level change	Policies developed; program elements institutionalised in the (health or other) system; program elements self-sustaining.	Reliability of policy measures; replication of process and impact effects.
Long-term health outcomes	Reduced morbidity, or reduced disease incidence; improved wellbeing or quality of life.	Validity of health outcomes or quality of life measures; predictive validity of intervention exposure on outcomes.
Diffusion and dissemination of program	Spread of effective program and resultant policy—process evaluation of dissemination.	Measures of dissemination and diffusion; reach of the program; uptake of program as proportion of eligible sites.

5.5 Summary

This chapter has described some of the important technical challenges in the evaluation of a program to generate evidence about effectiveness. First, the selection of people for the program is described. Then the steps of evaluation design, measurement issues and statistical testing are summarised. The better the research methods, the more confident we can be that the observed effects of a program were caused by the intervention and did not occur by chance, or were not due to other factors or influences. In all evaluation studies, there is an obligation to fully describe potential sources of bias, the sampling methods used and methods of data analysis in any report.

Measurement is a central part of impact evaluation. As well as the obvious impact or outcome measurements, relevant measures and indicators are needed at all stages of evaluation, from problem definition to outcomes assessment. The scope of health promotion measurement has expanded in recent decades from individual-level assessment of health beliefs and behaviours through to measures of concepts such as social capital, community empowerment and the attributes of coalitions and partnerships. In the latter areas, few measures exist and may need to be developed, to accurately assess health promotion actions, organisational or environmental outcomes and community-level social outcomes.

In summary, 'best practice' in health promotion evaluation requires continuous consideration of the optimal against the possible in evaluation design and measurement. No single approach represents the best evaluation design for all purposes. The best approach will vary depending on the context and setting of the program, the resources and time available, and the expressed needs of stakeholders for evidence of a program. In particular, as health promotion programs are larger and more complex (see Chapter 6), the potential for randomisation of participants and extensive validated assessments may become more limited.

References

Bauman AE, Sallis JF & Dzewaltowski DA et al. 2002, 'Towards a better understanding of the influences on physical activity: the role of determinants, correlates, causal variables, mediators, moderators and confounders', *American Journal of Preventative Medicine*, vol. 23 (2 Suppl), pp. 5–14.

Caria MP, Faggiano F & Bellocco R et al. 2011, 'Effects of a school-based prevention program on European adolescents patterns of alcohol use', *Journal of Adolescent Health*, vol. 48, no. 2, pp. 182–8.

Dumsha JZ, DiTomasso RA & Gomez FC et al. 2011, 'Changes in self-reported drinking behaviors among US teenagers associated with the introduction of flavored malt beverages: an interrupted time-series quasi-experiment', *Addiction Research and Theory*, vol. 19, no. 3, pp. 199–212.

Fledderus M, Bohlmeijer ET & Smit F et al. 2010, 'Mental health promotion as a new goal in public mental health care: a randomized controlled trial of an intervention enhancing psychological flexibility', *American Journal of Public Health*, vol. 100, no. 12, pp. 2372–8.

Killam WP, Tambatamba BC & Chintu N et al. 2010, 'Antiretroviral therapy in antenatal care to increase treatment initiation in HIV-infected pregnant women: a stepped-wedge evaluation', *AIDS*, vol. 24, no. 1, pp. 85–91.

Louis-Nance TR, Flournoy MW & Clinton KS et al. 2012, 'The Females Against Cancer Educational Series: a qualitative evaluation of mother/daughter knowledge and perceptions of human papilloma virus and its related cancers', *Journal of the National Medical Association*, vol. 104, nos 3–4, pp. 194–8.

McConnell D, Breitkreuz R & Savage A 2012, 'Independent evaluation of the Triple P Positive Parenting Program in family support service settings', *Child and Family Social Work*, vol. 17, no. 1, pp. 43–54.

Patel V, Weiss HA & Chowdhary N et al. 2010, 'Effectiveness of an intervention led by lay health counsellors for depressive and anxiety disorders in primary care in Goa, India (MANAS): a cluster randomised controlled trial', *Lancet*, vol. 376, no. 9758, pp. 2086–95.

Shelley D, Fahs M & Yerneni R et al. 2008, 'Effectiveness of tobacco control among Chinese Americans: a comparative analysis of policy approaches versus community-based programs', *Preventive Medicine*, vol. 47, no. 5, pp. 530–6.

Vadheim LM, Brewer KA & Kassner DR et al. 2010, 'Effectiveness of a lifestyle intervention program among persons at high risk for cardiovascular disease and diabetes in a rural community', *Journal of Rural Health*, vol. 26, no. 3, pp. 266–72.

Wing RR, Bahnson JL & Bray GA et al. 2010, 'Long-term effects of a lifestyle intervention on weight and cardiovascular risk factors in individuals with Type 2 diabetes Mellitus: four-year results of the LOOK AHEAD Trial', *Archives of Internal Medicine*, vol. 170, no. 17, pp. 1566–75.

6

Complex program evaluation

Many problems in public health and health promotion are not 'simple' and require long-term efforts to deliver a range of programs across settings to address complex issues. The science of **complex program evaluation (CPE)** is relatively young, but takes into account the complexity of the public health issue, and proposes evaluation of each component, as well as an overall summative assessment of progress. In CPE, process evaluation to monitor implementation, assess program reach and monitor adaptation are particularly important.

6.1 Background to complex program evaluation (CPE)

Chapter 5 presented evaluation designs and methods for simple interventions. In many cases, such projects may be short term, conducted within a 12-month funding cycle that includes the evaluation component. These interventions can sometimes have a population-wide focus, if they 'reach' a large and undifferentiated target population or community.

Moving from single-component interventions to CPE

Although single-component interventions can have population reach, typically they are conducted at a smaller scale, and are evaluated within well-defined populations and carefully managed environments; they may not provide evidence that is generalisable to a whole population. For example, a school-based intervention evaluated using a cluster randomised trial may be effective in encouraging healthier eating in schools, and may be evaluated using an optimal research design (see Chapter 5), but does not address the broader issues of food supply to adolescents or its marketing in stores and shopping malls. Much that may be achieved within the school intervention could be undermined by experiences outside of the targeted environment of the school. In many cases, single interventions may not be able to make a population-level difference without a more comprehensive suite of intervention components, strategies and partnerships.

This chapter is concerned with assessing the effects of more comprehensive efforts to promote health at the population level. These can be labelled 'complex public health programs'. These extend beyond single-component interventions, and are comprised of multiple components designed to influence a range of agencies, organisations and individuals to achieve sustainable population change. These complex programs are defined as 'interventions with several interacting elements aimed at whole populations or community settings… targeting any or all of individuals, settings, professionals or policy makers' (Craig et al. 2008).

Single-component interventions that can reach whole populations

Some population-scale interventions may be comprised of just a single component. This means that the intervention may have wide reach, but consists of only one intervention component. Examples of these include:

1. web-based behaviour change trials;
2. single-issue mass media campaigns;
3. specific environmental interventions.

In the first of these examples, a web-based trial might target smoking or a healthy diet, using web-based media and new media to deliver a standardised, theoretically defined behaviour change intervention to a potentially very large sample who choose to participate in the intervention. In the second example, a standalone mass media campaign might target condom usage and HIV prevention, communicated only through selective mass media targeting an at-risk population group. The third example might be a specific environmental intervention, such as building a new trail or walking route, and evaluating the impact of that single intervention on the physical activity levels of people living near the trail. All three examples could be discrete interventions, without additional or supportive components, that could be evaluated using the principles outlined in Chapter 5. Although interventions such as these may often occur in population health practice as discrete interventions, this may not be optimal; for example, the web intervention could be supplemented by additional individualised support; the mass media campaign should be supported by community mobilisation and by relevant policy and environmental changes; and the trail construction supported by local marketing, making these all more 'complex' interventions.

This chapter is concerned with more complex interventions, comprising multiple components and posing greater challenges for evaluation.

6.2   Complex public health interventions

Many public health interventions require more than just a single mode of intervention in order to reach and produce sustainable change in a whole population or target group. This is the newly developing science and practice of implementing and evaluating complex health promotion programs. The problem can sometimes be construed as an interconnected 'system', and 'systems approaches' may be needed to understanding complex health problems and planning effective solutions (Luke & Stamatakis 2012). This needs a different approach to evaluation, building on the research designs and methods described in Chapter 5, and adding elements to appraise an interacting set of community interventions and programs in order to understand effects in more complex real-world settings. The field of CPE is premised on the idea that the problems to be solved have multiple causes (*determinants*) at many levels, and the solutions required may involve multiple concurrent intervention components and strategies (Smith & Petticrew 2010).

The history of complex preventive programs at multiple levels dates back to the 1980s or earlier, and has been a part of health promotion program delivery for many years. Many initial comprehensive cardiovascular disease prevention trials followed the principles of complex programs, although mixed-method approaches to evaluation were less often applied. These programs included the Stanford Three and Five City Preventions programs, the community-wide heart disease prevention programs in Pawtucket and Minnesota, USA, the North Karelia project in Finland and Heartbeat Wales in the UK (Nutbeam et al. 1993). The subsequent health promotion frameworks developed through the 1986 Ottawa Charter, the evolution of environment and policy interventions for the prevention of chronic disease, and the more recent development of 'systems thinking' have all contributed to the field of CPE development. In essence, complex interventions are a 'program' of work, more than just a single 'project' evaluation, and require more sophisticated approaches to evaluation. One needs to define the components that summate to the overall program of work, specify the outcomes likely to be influenced from individual components and their combinations, identify how data are to be collected, and involve stakeholders in the planning and implementation of the complex program. A summary of the net effects, benefits and mechanisms of program activity is the 'summative' evaluation conducted at the end of the program, bringing together the multiple evaluation elements. The **summative evaluation** of complex programs is usually comprised of mixed methods, including both quantitative and qualitative methods and data collection.

A schema for planning complex interventions is shown in Figure 6.1 on page 92. This extends the planning process, logic model development and process and impact evaluation described in Chapters 2–5. The planning steps may not be linear; they include establishing what has been tried before, and identifying that effectiveness was not demonstrated or was confined to selected samples only (in other words, the evidence was not generalisable). Having decided that more complex, intersecting components are required, then planning processes, logic models and overall pre-program costing should be undertaken. In complex programs, the range of expected outcomes may not be linear, as different outcomes of different components may occur at different rates and in different settings, and evaluators must allow sufficient time for effects to be detected and measured. The complex program consists of multiple elements, and the logic model at the planning stage might consider the effects and sequencing of these different components. For example, a sexual-health program in UK schools was assessed in terms of initial changes to curriculums, to Education Department policies, to teachers' practices, as well as the target audience of adolescents (Henderson et al. 2007). These more complex forms of formative, process and impact evaluation are described in the rest of this chapter.

6.3   Formative and process evaluation for CPE

As with single-focus interventions, the planning and formative evaluation of a complex program of work starts with a review of the evidence and a theoretical framework (Figure 6.1). This builds on the logic models described in Chapter 3 and applied to single interventions in Chapters 4 and 5, but the frameworks are more complicated. Sometimes, there are too many diverse

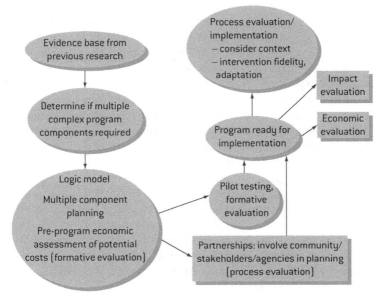

Figure 6.1 Complex interventions: planning and evaluation stages

causal factors to target all of them in a complex program. Thus, selected determinants, or selected components, are usually chosen for consideration and development. The theoretical underpinnings may include an integrated 'systems theory' approach, rather than only relying on individual or group behaviour change models.

A detailed evaluation plan should be developed, with objectives, proposed research methods and outcomes *for each component*. This makes the overall tasks of evaluation more complex, as each piece of the program will need consideration from an evaluation perspective. The time frame, methods of data collection and measures should be specified, so that the evaluation tasks, the accountable agencies or evaluators and their cost in personnel and resources will all be estimated at the outset. The intervention and all its components should be described, and expected changes identified, across all levels: changes in stakeholders, organisations, communities, environments, policy and individuals. Hypothetical economic modelling may be undertaken as an important part of program evaluation, to assess what the potential changes might mean in terms of intervention costs, system costs or community cost savings (Figure 6.1).

The next steps are assessing the feasibility of implementing the program, ensuring sufficient resources and staff to intervene at multiple levels, and considering the different settings (contexts) in which the intervention is to be delivered. Formative evaluation may include stakeholder and community consultation, and their participation in program component planning and development.

> *The process of community engagement in planning is challenging and time-consuming, but is important to assess the feasibility and likely community acceptance of the multiple components that are planned.*

A central part of CPE is carrying out thorough process evaluation, building on the evaluation procedures outlined in Chapters 3–5. Process evaluation will be required for all components, as well as an overall judgment across the whole program. Examples include:

- assessment of component *reach* (*intervention fidelity*): whether all schools made changes; whether all intervention components were implemented as planned;
- *context*: what local and external factors influenced uptake and program delivery;

- *acceptability* of the proposed changes;
- *sustainability* of the intervention components at medium to long-term follow-up.

Evaluating fidelity and adaptation

The degree of intervention 'flexibility' or adaptation that occurs in the field will vary from setting to setting, and a key evaluation task is to determine whether the fidelity of the intervention implementation is close enough to the original concept to be likely to achieve positive outcomes. This contrasts with single project interventions, where implementation is likely to be more standardised. There has been some debate on the issue of to what degree CPE implementation should be standardised across complex systems (Shiell et al. 2008), and whether evaluation efforts should focus on identifying the conditions that lead to better implementation, as a central task of CPE.

For example, in trying to deliver a complex program to several schools, there will be variation in delivery, resources, facilities and uptake. The evaluation question is concerned with assessing different aspects of program fidelity:

- To what extent is a policy to deliver a standard school-based or workplace intervention implemented across each of many regions?
- How different can an intervention be from that originally developed, and still be effective? For example, could the curriculum part be delivered in fewer sessions?
- What impact would an intervention have if the school canteen component was not implemented (as part of a hypothetical overall nutrition program)?
- Can a hypothetical planned six-session lifestyle change program or curriculum be as effective if delivered in only four sessions at some intervention sites?

These examples of evaluation questions are related to implementation in complex programs and need to be addressed at multiple levels. Process evaluation is central to building an understanding of why and how a program worked (or failed), which is instructive for future efforts in addressing the same problem. This information contributes to answering questions about whether the lack of an apparent effect was due to true ineffectiveness in a population, or to implementation failure (this is assessed by good process evaluation, described in Chapters 2 and 5).

6.4 Evaluation designs for complex programs

Evaluation designs for complex programs build on those described in previous chapters, and employ both qualitative and quantitative methods. In complex programs, multiple parallel and sequential evaluation tasks are needed, making evaluation planning a more comprehensive and demanding activity than in single intervention evaluations.

Impact evaluation is used to document clear achievement of the objectives of each program sub-component. These might include measures of community residents or school students or workplace employees at a defined baseline and at follow-up, questionnaires or surveys of managers, staff and stakeholders, and assessments of changes to policy and to the social and physical activity environments that are targeted. This extends the description of 'health promotion outcomes' presented in Chapter 1 (Figure 1.2), but here we point out that multiple outcomes may need to be concurrently assessed in the large evaluation tasks of assessing one complex program. In some CPEs, evaluation may only occur at an organisational or community level, without individual-level measurement, and in others, evaluation will occur at multiple levels.

Research designs build on those in Chapter 5, with ideal CPEs using randomised or cluster randomised designs (recommended by Craig et al. 2008; Macintyre & Petticrew 2000). However, the complexity of real-world interventions (multiple, phased interventions across a whole population) may make a randomised trial design impractical if not impossible. Non-randomised designs may be more likely when policy-makers are reluctant to randomise regions or sites, or when other considerations dictate where the intervention should be delivered first. Checklists of 'good practice' criteria for non-randomised trial designs have been developed (see Appendix 5).

In CPEs, other kinds of research designs may be useful, for example, where an intervention involves phased rollout of the intervention across sites (stepped-wedge design), or preference trials. A stepped-wedge design may be useful where there is a strong policy interest in implementing a program, but its effectiveness is not known; in many such situations, there are insufficient resources for the program to be universally provided, so a rollout over time across different regions is proposed, and rollout can occur according to a randomisation schedule (see Chapter 5). Quasi-experimental designs are commonly used, with program and comparison regions, and if carefully planned, can provide useful evidence of program effects (Bonell et al. 2011).

In addition to research designs that assess primary outcomes, other methods may be used in process evaluation of key program components. These can be conceptualised as process evaluations of:

1. key public health professionals, stakeholders and policy-makers' engagement;
2. process evaluations of the implementation of programs (delivery, reach, fidelity);
3. process evaluation of the implementation of policies or construction of facilities (changes to the built environment).

For example, pre–post quantitative or qualitative surveys may be delivered to stakeholders, but audits or other implementation measures used to assess changes to the environments or adoption of policies. Different methods of data collection, such as qualitative interviews, focus groups or observations, can be triangulated with quantitative information collected elsewhere, to corroborate or refute evaluation findings.

The measures used will also be at multiple levels, including individual-level change in awareness, beliefs or behaviours, changes in professional practice, in organisation-level policy implementation, in the physical or social environments in which the intervention took place, or in the community-level policy. This extends the discussion of measurement in Chapter 5, since multiple levels and types of measurement are usually required in CPEs. The intersecting elements of the program might target change at these different levels, and the challenge in evaluation is to measure more than just individual-level change. The research design and measurement tasks summate to a set of mixed-method 'sub-evaluations' within the overall CPE.

Use of population surveillance

In some situations, instead of specific individual program surveys or interviews, it may be possible to use overarching population surveillance to evaluate complex programs. This is possible also in evaluating long-term single interventions, but may be more usual in assessing CPEs, given the longer time frames for implementing multiple program components. For example, many regions or nations collect annual representative population health surveys, and these can be used to track changes in the population in a standardised way and over several years following the intervention, and assess the net sum of the complex program components on a single indicator, such as smoking rates or falls in a community. This method is often used, but may have insufficient sample size to assess intervention effects in different regions, where process evaluation data have shown differential levels of program implementation.

Whether to use or adapt population surveillance to the evaluation of CPEs can be determined by assessing costs, the hypothesised time frame for assessing individual-level changes, and the need to monitor the sustainability of initial gains. Specific questions relevant to evaluation may be integrated into routine population surveys, if they can be included in a timely manner, and repeated over multiple years in these surveillance systems.

Beyond the sub-components of formative, process and impact evaluations, these complex programs need an overview evaluation, often described as a summative evaluation. This considers data from different sources and collected using diverse methods, and assesses an overall picture of success. Here, data from different information sources are examined, to see if the findings corroborate each other; this is known as triangulation of data. For example, consider an integrated multi-site sun-protection intervention aimed at reducing sun exposure among school-age children:

- Was the policy implemented the same way across regions (high fidelity and reach)?
- Did the school education modules about sun protection have the same impact in different schools?
- Did the mass media campaign targeting parents of young children reach all socioeconomic groups in the region?
- Did qualitative interviews with groups of parents from diverse cultural backgrounds indicate that they understood the sun-protection messages in the same way?
- Did sun-protection practices change over time?

These components may have been part of one large-scale program, but if the evaluations of sub-components point in the same direction (well implemented in communities; school students responded similarly; different groups of parents all aware of the initiative), then this is a good example of 'triangulation' of the results, indicating a successful overall or 'summative' evaluation of this complex program. Summative evaluation is more difficult if the different components show effects in different directions, or if some components did not work or reach anticipated populations; then summative evaluation becomes a qualitative 'impression', whether the 'net sum' of effective components is likely to improve population health, or not.

6.5 Challenges in conducting CPEs

The community-wide 'system' in which CPEs are required poses challenges to evaluation theory and practice. The three main issues on evaluating complex programs relate to:

- program planning and logic;
- implementation;
- technical, analytical issues.

First, there needs to be flexibility in the evaluation plan, as the implementation of diverse intervention components may not follow a logic model as clearly as a single-component intervention does. There may be other concurrent programs or policies at work in parts of the 'system' addressing the same health issue, and it may not be possible to disentangle the causal effects of individual components. The management and conduct of complex programs are difficult, and a team or partnership group with representation from different agencies may be required to manage and coordinate efforts. Efforts to scale the program to achieve real population-wide effects are difficult to achieve. For example, there may be delays in some regions in the implementation of a particular screening or immunisation schedule as part of an overall prevention program. Similarly, a program to reduce the consumption of sweetened drinks in a community could be implemented and evaluated in different ways; for example, vending machines might be phased out, but only in 10 of 30 schools in the region; workplace policies might be ignored in half of workplace canteens; community health staff might be unaware of the program; and only half of the shops or stores might implement the policy to replace high-calorie beverages with lower calorie options.

Understanding the delivery and implementation mechanisms is important for understanding complex programs and may explain the observed quantitative impact. For this reason, it is essential to carry out high-quality process evaluations in CPE.

Impact and outcome data are often collected, but sufficient time is needed between the program delivery and the time required for complex changes to become evident. If documenting program impact is considered achievable, or is politically necessary, then attention to research design is important. However, caution must be exercised in expecting results from complex programs in the short term, and sufficient time, often a number of years, may be required to develop and implement multiple intervention components across a whole population (this builds on the timescale referred to in Chapter 1, Figure 1.3).

For quantitative data in CPEs, specialised analytic techniques may be needed, including statistical methods for analysing longitudinal data, approaches to analysing multi-level data, and obtaining validated measurements of the diverse range of psychosocial, behavioural and organisational outcomes that might be assessed. Collecting information on program costs and calculating cost-effectiveness may be useful in deciding if a complex intervention is worthwhile, as these complex interventions are long-term investments in public health, and usually require substantial resources and commitment of staff.

Example of a hypothetical CPE

To illustrate this, a hypothetical example of a school-based intervention to reduce childhood obesity across an entire community is used as a case study (see Box 6.1). In this school example, there is teacher training (one intervention component), resource delivery (another component), student access and participation in the curriculum, and delivery of the new curriculum components as intended. In many CPEs, there will be individual outcomes; professional or stakeholder evaluation; and context/system/environment evaluation components. This may need a logic model to be developed, to identify all the programmatic inputs and expected outcomes.

Box 6.1 A hypothetical complex school-led intervention to reduce childhood obesity

The primary goal of this school-based program might be (1) to reduce childhood obesity among primary-school children, with a number of secondary goals of improving (2) schools' food supply to children; (3) physical education in schools; and (4) the home environment of students regarding nutrition and physical activity.

Each of these components (or parts) needs an evaluation itself, consistent with the overall and sub-component program goals. For example, part 1 might be assessed by a cluster randomised controlled trial, allocating some schools to the intervention and others as controls; objective measures of weight, diet and physical activity among students before the program (say, at year 3 of school), and again after the program four years later. Parts 2 and 3 may need process evaluation: were the school food service innovations introduced, and was the physical education curriculum implemented and delivered to all students? In addition, qualitative interviews with teachers, canteen staff and other stakeholders may provide different perspectives on the program implementation, and help to explain or understand the primary outcome results. Part 4 of the evaluation might involve strategies with parents' attitudes to and usage of fast food or sugar-sweetened drinks, or to increase local sports club or facility usage. These program components need many overlapping evaluation elements, including parental surveys, qualitative interviews and environmental audits over time.

Using a logic model, and combining information from each evaluation task, a summary of the effects and explanations for the whole program can be generated, using information collected in each sub-evaluation.

In the example in Box 6.1, four components were evaluated, but more are possible in the real world, and decisions made in the logic-model planning phase determine which parts require which levels of evaluation. In addition, economic models of the cost and effectiveness of this kind of complex intervention is often warranted (see Appendix 4 for brief details of economic evaluation methods). Where different parts of an evaluation or different methods are used to examine similar phenomena, data triangulation (described above) will be very useful; if parts 2, 3 and 4 show positive results, then it would be expected that the primary outcome would also show results in the expected direction, with improvements in physical activity, health dietary choices and less weight gain in intervention schools compared to control schools.

Good examples of CPE show the best possible scientific rigour in impact evaluation, and a range of appropriate and often mixed methods across formative and process evaluation components, in order to understand the program impact results and explain why and where an intervention component worked or did not work, which is important for subsequent CPE efforts in this area. Examples from three different countries are shown in Table 6.1, targeting mental health in the elderly in Holland, childhood disease in Bangladesh, and lifestyle risks in deprived neighbourhoods in the UK. These examples illustrate the diversity of measurement, design and intervention complexity used in CPE. Note that, before a CPE paper is published, several additional studies are often sought, reporting formative, qualitative, process and impact evaluation information, and subsequent papers reporting longer term maintenance data.

Table 6.1 Published examples of CPEs showing 'complexity' in formative, process and impact evaluation

Author (year) and project	Formative evaluation (FE) and process evaluation (PE)	Impact evaluation/ intervention design	Issues around 'complexity'
de Vlaming et al. (2010): healthy ageing in a Dutch community	FE: based on Dutch policy for 'healthy ageing'; logic model designed; partnerships formed; community analyses undertaken, 18 months. PE: sequenced interventions, two years, assessed reach, feasibility and acceptance.	Quasi-experimental design, one intervention and one control community. Focus on measures of loneliness and social connections; careful attention to sample size and measures used in surveys.	Multiple components including a campaign to increase awareness; social networking using older adult services and community; link to local government initiatives.

Author (year) and project	Formative evaluation (FE) and process evaluation (PE)	Impact evaluation/ intervention design	Issues around 'complexity'
Arifeen et al. (2009): local communities in Bangladesh	Six-year program of work to improve early childhood health, through improving housing, health literacy in the community, improving guideline-based healthcare delivery, preventive practices for mothers.	Cluster RCT of 20 healthcare facilities in Bangladesh. Measures included housing, village attributes, healthcare skills, healthcare delivery mechanisms, preventive practices, disease incidence, childhood mortality.	Multiple measures, to assess different components of the overall program; program elements were integrated to improve different determinants of early childhood ill health, ranging from breastfeeding rates, domestic hygiene and clinical care. Comparison regions also improved, due to national immunisation, family planning, child health and nutritional guidelines.
Wall (2009): Well London project (see www.welllondon.org.uk)	Four-year program in 20 deprived neighbourhoods in London; interventions focused on healthy lifestyle and mental health. Collaboration of local government, local health authorities, other agencies and NGOs.	Cluster RCT, 10 intervention and 10 control neighbourhoods. Population surveys (100/cluster). Qualitative studies in each intervention area, intervention mapping (IM), interviews with project team and community. Routine surveillance data collections from health, crime, education and other sectors. Environment and policy audits.	Broad intersectoral health promotion partnerships formed into a coalition. Evaluation goals focused on effectiveness and cost-effectiveness analyses. Included adolescent component and adolescent measurement. Multiple data sets; an attempt at 'system-wide' assessment.

6.6 Summary

Single-component interventions may be insufficient to address the determinants of public health problems, and hence a more multi-layered program of work, over a more prolonged time period, may be required. Complex programs, comprised of multiple components and different levels, are often required to tackle difficult problems. These require CPE approaches, including multiple evaluation elements, mixed qualitative and quantitative techniques, and a summative evaluation at the end of the program, in order to summarise effects, strengths and weaknesses of the proposed efforts. These are long-term, resource-intensive programs of work, and evaluation efforts need to be equally sophisticated, at multiple levels and using high-quality process and impact evaluation to assess program results. The best possible evaluation methods should be applied to these programs, which may include a mixture of high levels of scientific rigour as well as qualitative information from participants, stakeholders and program delivery staff to identify reasons for program success and failure. The science and art of CPE is developing rapidly, but requires intensive multidisciplinary evaluation expertise and resources.

References

Arifeen SE, Hoque DME & Akter T et al. 2009, 'Effect of the Integrated Management of Childhood Illness strategy on childhood mortality and nutrition in a rural area in Bangladesh: a cluster randomised trial', *Lancet*, vol. 374, no. 9687, pp. 393–403.

Bonell CP, Hargreaves J & Cousens S et al. 2011, 'Alternatives to randomisation in the evaluation of public health interventions: design challenges and solutions', *Journal of Epidemiology and Community Health*, vol. 65, no. 7, pp. 582–7.

Craig P, Dieppe P & Macintyre S et al. 2008, 'Developing and evaluating complex interventions: the new Medical Research Council guidance', *British Medical Journal*, vol. 337, no. 7676.

de Vlaming R, Haveman-Nies A, van't Veer P, de Groot L 2010, 'Evaluation design for a complex intervention program targeting loneliness in non-institutionalized elderly Dutch people', *BMC Public Health*, vol. 10, no. 552.

Des Jarlais DC, Lyles C & Crepaz N et al. 2004, 'Improving the reporting quality of nonrandomized evaluations of behavioral and public health interventions: the TREND statement', *American Journal of Public Health*, vol. 94, no. 3, pp. 361–6.

Henderson M, Wight D & Raab GM et al. 2007, 'Impact of a theoretically based sex education programme (SHARE) delivered by teachers on NHS registered conceptions and terminations: final results of cluster randomised trial', *British Medical Journal*, vol. 334, no. 133.

Luke DA & Stamatakis KA 2012, 'Systems science methods in public health: dynamics, networks, and agents', *Annual Review of Public Health*, vol. 33, pp. 357–76.

Macintyre S & Petticrew M 2000, 'Good intentions and received wisdom are not enough', *Journal of Epidemiology and Community Health*, vol. 54, no. 11, pp. 802–3.

Nutbeam D, Smith C & Murphy S et al. 1993, 'Maintaining evaluation designs in long-term community-based health promotion programs: Heartbeat Wales case-study', *Journal of Epidemiology and Community Health*, vol. 47, no. 2, pp. 127–33.

Shiell A, Hawe P & Gold L 2008, 'Complex interventions or complex systems? Implications for health economic evaluation', *British Medical Journal*, vol. 336, no. 7656, pp. 1281–3.

Smith RD & Petticrew M 2010, 'Public health evaluation in the twenty-first century: time to see the wood as well as the trees', *Journal of Public Health*, vol. 32, no. 1, pp. 2–7.

Wall M, Hayes R & Moore D et al. 2009, 'Evaluation of community-level interventions to address social and structural determinants of health: a cluster randomised controlled trial', *BMC Public Health*, vol. 9, no. 207.

Evaluation methods for program replication, dissemination and institutionalisation

Public health change requires reaching large proportions of the population with an intervention. This chapter is concerned with evaluation of efforts to test established interventions in new groups (*replication studies*) and to scale them up to even larger populations (*dissemination*). The evaluation focus is on increasing the emphasis on process evaluation, to understand implementation of interventions at a larger scale.

This chapter is concerned with the stages of program replication, dissemination and institutionalisation, beyond the initial testing of whether a program works. This is a new area of evaluation and is fundamental to assessing the significance of public health programs. Chapters 5 and 6 described the evaluation of individual and complex public health interventions and programs, identifying the evaluation design options and summarising important technical issues. Many published studies are conducted in small or selected samples and, if evaluated well, provide a good indication of whether the program works in certain conditions with certain populations. Through the evaluation process, some health promotion interventions are found to be effective, affordable and well-implemented; others would not meet these criteria.

The next public health challenge is to scale up a successful project in order to reach a broader population level. The stages of replication or demonstration are based on the need to deliver interventions and programs to larger and more representative groups. The concept of 'scaling up' is defined as the 'ability of a health intervention shown to be efficacious on a small scale and/or under controlled conditions to be expanded under real-world conditions to reach a greater proportion of the eligible population, while retaining effectiveness' (Milat 2011). This covers both intervention demonstration (replication studies, stage 4 in Figure 2.1, Chapter 2) if they are conducted in larger samples and the next stage, intervention dissemination (stage 5, Figure 2.1, Chapter 2) when interventions are applied to whole populations.

Finally, the last stage, institutionalisation, is reached, where the program becomes incorporated into the routine work of public health agencies or government departments.

Repeated and consistently observed intervention effects will assist health authorities and funders in identifying which programs are suitable for policy support and large-scale dissemination and even institutionalisation. Alternatively, it is risky and unwise to base a policy decision to scale up a program and commit significant funding on evidence derived from one evaluation study conducted at one point in time in one setting, especially if results are equivocal or the effects are small. This is true even if the area is a key priority area and evidence is scarce.

> *The results of negative evaluations are also important, but often ignored; programs shown repeatedly not to be effective should not be considered for dissemination.*

7.1 Stages in assessing the significance of programs

This chapter describes three stages:
1. replication;
2. dissemination;
3. institutionalisation.

The first stage tests interventions in new and different populations, to examine whether they produce similar effects; the second scales up programs to a larger population level, to disseminate the effective program widely and assess whether it can be scaled up; and the third makes a program part of routine service delivery or public health, institutionalising the program within the 'system'. These stages are shown conceptually in Figure 7.1 on page 106, with increasing numbers in the target population exposed to and engaging with the intervention. Note that the initial efficacy or evidence-generating study is shown as a diamond in the far left-hand corner of the figure; with intervention demonstration (replication) studies, the samples reached are usually larger and more representative. The next stage, testing the intervention in dissemination studies, reaches large segments of the population, shown as rectangular segments in Figure 7.1. The final stage of institutionalisation is where the whole population is reached, shown as universal background shading, with all people exposed to the initiative.

The three stages may seem obvious, but after years of working on trying to find solutions to public health problems, practitioners and researchers

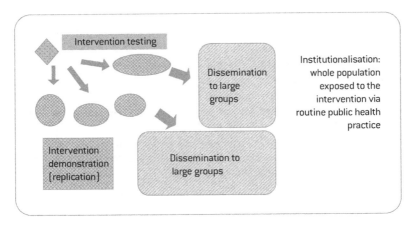

Figure 7.1 Stages in scaling up interventions to achieve population health

may lose sight of the population-wide goal the stages are seeking to achieve. One of the problems with much of the published 'evidence' is that it is usually researcher-initiated, focused on demonstrating that something works in carefully managed conditions. This is important in establishing the feasibility of an intervention, but does not of itself produce population health benefits. We need more practice-based, relevant 'evidence' that might make a population difference and is feasible within available (constrained) resources and compatible with current service delivery (Green & Glasgow 2006). This requires new modes of scaled-up program delivery, with concomitant new approaches to evaluation that will clearly inform policy-makers regarding interventions (Wilson et al. 2010).

The links between evidence generation and making a population difference are illustrated in Figure 7.2. The left-hand side of the figure shows 'researcher-driven' approaches, from obtaining research funding to 'evidence generation', the stage of assessing effectiveness. This illustrates the funding drivers that determine the kinds of research that is conducted and the kinds of evidence that are generated. Researchers are influenced by national and local research priorities and have the tasks of developing and testing specific interventions in selected samples. The best research methods (ideally using formative, process and impact evaluation methods) are sought, to produce the highest scientific quality of evidence. There may be a cycle of refining evidence, testing alternative interventions, but again these are usually in small-scale or selected samples.

If the evidence base is to be more population-relevant, then interventions and their evaluation need to be scaled up. This is shown on the right-hand side of Figure 7.2, providing information of particular relevance to practice

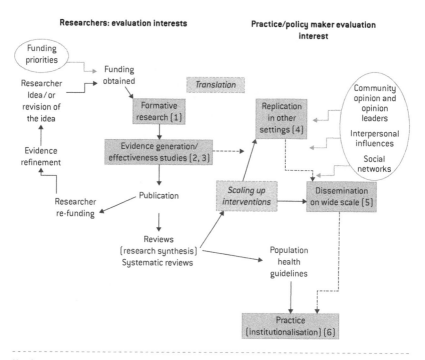

Numbers represent stages, as shown in the model in Chapter 2, Figure 2.1.

Figure 7.2 Conceptual framework for research replication and dissemination

and policy-makers. These stages include replication research on interventions in new settings and with new populations and disseminating interventions to whole regions, or finally to be adopted at a system level and institutionalised in public health practice.

In addition, the process includes the adoption and dissemination of evidence and information to policy- and decision-makers, a process that we describe as 'knowledge translation' (Rychetnik et al. 2012), summarised in Box 7.1 on page 108. This process precedes, or is concurrent with, efforts at replication and dissemination of evidence, and often requires their support to plan and implement dissemination studies.

7.2 Replication (intervention demonstration)

The first purpose of replication is to confirm the scientific findings of program effectiveness and to assess whether similar effects are found when the intervention is conducted in different populations. The effects observed in

Box 7.1 Research translation

The concept of 'research translation' is often confused with the actual scaling up of interventions. Strictly, we define 'research translation' as the process of working with the public health system and with policy-makers to increase the acceptance of evidence-based solutions and to create the conditions for scaling up interventions (Rychetnik et al. 2012); this is fundamental to garnering the support and resources for implementing interventions at a larger scale and applying research evidence to more generalisable population settings. This is sometimes carried out through research syntheses, which are then translated as public health 'guidelines' by the relevant government departments (see Figure 7.2). This step is necessary to, but separate from, the process for implementing a program across a large region. It is necessary to enable policy support, funding, redeployment of staff and the development of evaluation and monitoring frameworks for replication and dissemination work.

the original study may not be easily repeatable, as they may have been due to specific characteristics in the samples used in the initial study, for example, the level of commitment among stakeholders; enthusiastic and well-organised program delivery; or the unique characteristics of the setting in which the initial evaluation study was conducted. Often, the initial study uses motivated volunteers or socially and educationally advantaged groups with high levels of health literacy, so that the effects and outcomes seen in these groups are not generalisable.

There is an important but subtle difference between *repetition* and *replication*. *Repetition* tests a slightly different program, a slightly varied intervention or a different theoretical approach to facilitating change, but in essentially similar samples to the original. This approach is typical in the published literature, where minor variants on an intervention are tested in essentially similar groups of people. Repetitive studies also focus on 'efficacy testing' as the main research goal. By contrast, *replication* implies testing and evaluation of an already efficacious intervention in quite different groups of people and/or diverse contexts, which tests the intervention in circumstances that are closer to real life. For these reasons, replication studies place a much stronger emphasis on process evaluation, on assessing the degree of implementation, program fidelity and participant acceptance of the intervention in these new populations and settings.

There are two key questions for evaluation at this stage:

- Can the intervention *outcomes* be replicated in similar and in dissimilar settings, or will the individual-level and organisational-level outcomes vary in different settings and populations? This requires a focus on measuring the same outcomes as observed in the original intervention.

- Can the intervention *implementation* be replicated in diverse settings? This requires process evaluation, assessing whether delivery of the intervention is similarly feasible, delivered in the same way and accepted in diverse settings and groups.

The need for further replication studies becomes obvious when individual effectiveness studies are examined more closely. For example, an initial work site health promotion intervention might have been tested within a single work site and shown to be effective in producing a range of lifestyle risk-factor improvements or reduced stress or other positive outcomes. What may not be so evident from the study results is that the work site contained a much higher proportion of white-collar workers and that the management was highly supportive of the program implementation. In such circumstances, it is essential to examine whether these same effects would be found in other work sites with higher proportions of blue-collar workers, or with different age/gender distributions, different shift working hours among employees, across multiple sites and with less obvious management support.

Replication increases confidence that the observed effects are real and that this level of change in outcomes might be achieved elsewhere or, in other words, is generalisable to different populations and settings. The number of replications or settings is not fixed; this depends on the policy priorities in the region or country, but at least one replication of a program in a different setting should be conducted before wider dissemination of a program is considered.

Evaluation methods in replication studies

Evaluation methods for replication are slightly different to those in the initial efficacy study. It is essential that replication studies use identical outcome measures, so that effects are comparable. The evaluation designs for replication studies might use designs described in Chapter 5, such as quasi-experimental or controlled trials, but could utilise 'before–after' designs. The latter design is more acceptable in replication studies because the effect size (i.e. the change in the target outcomes) is already established from the original efficacy trial. The settings for replication are not necessarily randomly sampled. Indeed, in replication studies purposive sampling to maximise the diversity of settings for examination might be most useful.

Conducting good process evaluation is the central evaluation task in replication studies. We need to identify if the program can be implemented as intended in different settings, or whether it will require adaptation in different contexts to produce the same effects as the original trial. These contextual differences may be due to different levels of resourcing and management support or different characteristics of program participants. It is important to ask how much adaptation is needed and whether the intervention produces similar effects with different degrees of adaptation of implementation. This type of information is essential for health practitioners who have responsibility for implementing programs.

> *If the program implementation cannot be replicated (with adaptation as necessary) in different circumstances, then further implementation of the program in different sites would not yield the same results as the original program.*

Process evaluation in the replication phase helps to identify effective mechanisms for conducting the intervention in different groups and settings. Examples are shown in Table 7.1, where the shaded examples 1–4 in the upper half of the table demonstrate replication testing in larger samples (1), in a socially disadvantaged region (2), in multiple local districts (3) and assessing program delivery in additional settings (4). This kind of evaluation information is useful for program planners and policy-makers, to indicate whether the program is ready for the next stage, large-scale dissemination.

Table 7.1 Replication and dissemination examples

Example	Author (year)	Intervention	Dissemination
Replication studies			
1	Borawski et al. (2009)	HIV prevention (teenagers).	Cluster RCT. Replication in larger sample (no effect on sexual behaviour).
2	Vidrine et al. (2010)	Tobacco cessation with Quitline (adapted).	Testing Quitline usefulness in disadvantaged region (Texas).
3	Hooker et al. (2005) (A)	Existing CHAMPS program to increase physical activity in elderly.	Replication of CHAMPS in 13 local agencies (A); testing in socially disadvantaged regions (B).
4	Stewart et al. (2006) (B)		

Example	Author (year)	Intervention	Dissemination
Dissemination studies			
5	Layne et al. (2008)	Strength training for older US adults 2005–6.	Process evaluation of #classes established, #leaders, #older adults attending (N=2217).
6	Dunton et al. (2009)	Physical activity and nutrition program in Californian middle schools.	Assessed state-wide 50% reach (240 000 students), sample of students and teachers surveyed good implementation, ↑ PA, ↓ sweets.
7	Manfredi et al. (2011)	US practice guidelines for smoking cessation.	Three levels of dissemination of practice guidelines to clinics; assessed program fidelity, interventions received and used.
8	Reynolds et al. (2012)	Sun-protection behaviour in ski fields, 'Go Sun Smart'.	Dissemination testing in 68 ski fields in North America, tested two different dissemination strategies.

Replication studies are not funded as often as efficacy trials because the need for this stage is not always clear to academic research funders, or to policy-makers. Frustratingly, evidence generated from efficacy studies are often used by policy-makers as sufficient for widespread dissemination. Without an understanding of the implementation challenges faced in 'real-world' conditions, a program is less likely to be successfully disseminated and less likely to produce the intended outcomes when disseminated widely.

7.3 Dissemination

If a program can be successfully replicated, it can be considered for wider dissemination across systems, regions or indeed across a whole country. Note that dissemination is an active process and needs to be distinguished from diffusion (see Box 7.2 on page 112). Intervention dissemination (stage 5, Figure 2.1 in Chapter 2) is an intentional process of achieving the maximum uptake of effective and feasible interventions into a community. Effective dissemination depends on original evidence of effectiveness (stage 3 effectiveness studies) and evidence of adaptable implementation in diverse

Box 7.2 Comparison of 'dissemination' with the process of 'diffusion'

Dissemination is an active process, where the investigators invest efforts and resources to encourage update and utilisation of the program. By contrast, 'diffusion' is a more passive process, where a program, skill or attribute is gradually adopted by a community, at a variable speed, depending on local awareness and interest. Some communities or individuals will adopt a new idea more quickly and this will be facilitated by system factors and individual factors (especially education). In practice, there may be a component of adoption both in response to media reports and publicity (diffusion) and in response to active provision of programs (dissemination), which may occur concurrently, blurring the exact reasons for adoption. Careful evaluation (for example, asking people where they heard about the new program) can help distinguish these two processes. Further, adoption research can identify regions that are slower to take up new programs and identify areas of greater need for investment and effort.

situations (stage 4 replication studies), and will need continuing commitment from decision-makers and funders. In the latter case this may require supportive policy to enable the distribution of the program and to provide resources to enable the widespread distribution of a program across a community.

Dissemination is the process of actively scaling up an intervention to reach a much larger region or population (Green et al. 2009). An intervention can be scaled up to reach more individuals, more organisations, professionals or communities. A scaled-up intervention may have greater 'external validity', as it is reaching a whole population or more representative sample and thus the results are of population-level relevance, but will require much greater investment and resources.

The research methods for understanding dissemination were pioneered by Everett Rogers, who developed a framework for 'diffusion of innovation interventions' (described in Green et al. 2009). He identified that programs were more effectively disseminated if target populations and professionals perceived them as more advantageous compared to current actions; if they could be trialled by people or organisations adopting them; if they were compatible with existing practice; and if they were simple. These factors, as well as effectiveness, affordability, feasibility and simplicity (Green et al. 2009) are key factors influencing a decision on whether to disseminate a program.

In addition, there needs to be a population-wide system through which the innovation could be disseminated (Rabin et al. 2008). Some form of delivery system is a key part of the practice of dissemination and assessing it is an important part of evaluation. For more detailed discussion of this, see Brownson et al. (2012).

When contemplating the dissemination of an intervention, new formative evaluation may be necessary: are the communities and systems ready for the scaled-up intervention to be delivered to them? The questions are again formative, assessing community capacity and resources as prerequisites for scaling up an intervention. Then once the decision is made and resources garnered, the ongoing dissemination research is based heavily on process evaluation, particularly on evaluating the uptake and the sustainability of the intervention in the target population. Examples of the kinds of evaluation methods required build on process evaluation components (in Chapter 3), but add in systems-level evaluation. Since multi-component interventions may be adapted, interpreted and delivered differently across a whole population, an understanding of complex systems-level evaluation is useful here. This requires a 'best processes' approach (Trickett et al. 2011) rather than a 'best practice' approach, the latter defined only in terms of research excellence attributes (see Chapter 5).

The systems approach, involving the interaction of interventions, processes and settings, requires more flexible evaluation methods across the relevant sets of environments.

The discipline of dissemination research and evaluation is still in development, but the list below contains examples of some evaluation approaches:

1. Formative evaluation before dissemination, including measures of the 'political engagement' of key individuals, stakeholders and organisations; provision of required resources; and community readiness.

2. Process evaluation measures, including the proportion of the target population reached; number of settings adopting the intervention; the adaptability and flexibility of the intervention actually implemented and delivered; and techniques such as network analysis, which may help to define the spread or reach of program components.

3. Community-level measures, including changes in social norms, system delivery factors, and supportive changes to the environment; and policies for, and maintenance of, supportive partnerships.

4. Measures of intervention mediators and moderators, identifying which factors sustain and enhance the intervention directly and under

which sets of conditions or circumstances the overall intervention is best or most effectively delivered; network analysis may also help to define the spread or reach of program components. The next step in evaluation is to demonstrate the impact and costs of disseminated programs. A central evaluation purpose is to demonstrate that the effects of the disseminated program are not too different from those of the original trials, for example, when a less intensive intervention is all that can be realistically delivered in field conditions. Research designs may be 'pre–post' assessment, in subgroups of the whole population, to assess whether the impact is similar to that obtained in the initial evidence-generating studies. Other evaluation tasks are to document the inputs (costs and staffing required), track implementation (presence of consistent planning approaches and logic models in each setting) and develop tools for continuous tracking and monitoring of reach and impact.

Examples of dissemination research are shown in examples 5–8 in Table 7.1, which illustrate the indicators of dissemination and also the research tasks, testing different modes of disseminating preventive programs.

7.4   Institutionalisation

The last stage in the program development and evaluation process (stage 6 in Figure 2.1, Chapter 2) concerns the monitoring of a program that has been widely disseminated and has become part of routine public health service delivery. This stage of evaluation is primarily concerned with quality control and long-term monitoring and surveillance of outcomes at a population level. This applies in a situation where a program has been successfully disseminated into a community and has established policy support and funding mechanisms and continuing community support.

Examples of institutionalised programs are those accepted as needed across the population, delivered over many years and sustained by the public health or other systems. These might range from 'quitlines' offering telephone-based tobacco cessation counselling, universally available in many countries, and childhood immunisation programs. At this stage, a project has become integrated into the long-term functions of the host agency or organisation.

Assessing and monitoring successful institutionalisation may involve:

■   regular population monitoring to assess maintenance of the specific outcomes that are targeted, such as individual behaviours;

■   monitoring of continuing community engagement and support for the intervention, for example, participation rates and public opinion;

■ process evaluation to examine the extent to which defined elements of the program are consistently delivered as intended (quality control);

■ continued consideration of the relationship between the cost of a program and its population health benefits.

Evaluation of institutionalised programs is based on routine population surveillance and service quality control. In many regions, there are representative population health surveys, to which specific health promotion questions can be added. These surveys monitor trends in community beliefs about, and perceptions of, health issues and health behaviours. Trend data can be accumulated to demonstrate population effects over time, or to demonstrate a reversal in program effects if the program's hold or reach weakens and program adherence declines over time. This information is acquired in the background and is linked to routine surveys, not specifically conducted for monitoring the institutionalisation of a program. This set of research tasks is also relevant for monitoring the implementation of national programs or initiatives and health promotion guidelines.

. A second component could include monitoring of representative or leading community stakeholders, coalitions and taskforces, to assess their ongoing support for the program. This can be in the form of surveys, qualitative interviews or policy analysis to assess the progress towards institutional acceptance and implementation from a decision-maker and resource allocation perspective.

Process evaluation remains central in stage 6 evaluation (see Chapter 2, Figure 2.1) and will require resources and effort. Implementation across many sites requires quality control, to make sure that the programs delivered have enough elements of the original program to remain effective. These evaluation tasks can assist decision-makers in the ongoing maintenance of established programs. Hypothetical examples of monitoring tasks for institutionalised programs are shown in Box 7.3.

Box 7.3 Examples of policy and environment evaluation tasks for institutionalised programs

1. Monitoring of public health services and other sector program delivery:
   a. for physical activity in children: are established physical education programs continuing to be delivered by the education sector to all schools?
   b. for illicit drug harm-reduction: are established needle and syringe exchange programs still widely available in the health system? Are they accessed by those that need them? Are they available in different regions/outreach clinics?

(continued)

Box 7.3 *continued*

   c. for cancer prevention: are evidence-based cancer screening services accessed by all at-risk target population groups?

   d. for equity and access: do effective adolescent drug and alcohol programs reach all marginalised and disadvantaged youth?

   e. for chronic disease management: are self-management programs for chronic illness available to all eligible individuals (for example, asthma, diabetes or arthritis education and management programs; cardiac rehabilitation programs)?

2. Monitoring of policy, and maintenance and adherence in the community:

   a. for tobacco control: are policies, for example, restricting tobacco sales to minors or plain packaging of cigarettes, being adhered to by shop owners and stores?

   b. for healthy nutrition: are policies about advertising of unhealthy foods or beverages to children being adhered to?

   c. for urbanisation and health, healthy cities: are established health-promoting urban development policies with a health impact being complied with?

   d. for HIV/sexually transmitted infection (STI) prevention: as part of an institutionalised 'safe sex' campaign, are condoms freely available from a range of outlets in the community?

7.5 Summary

This chapter has focused on the different evaluation tasks and measures for the replication, dissemination and institutionalisation of health promotion programs. In testing the efficacy of innovative interventions, careful attention to evaluation design, measures and internal validity is needed, to increase confidence that the observed effects were caused by the intervention and did not occur by chance, or because of other factors or influences.

Once an intervention has been demonstrated to be effective, the evaluation task is far from over. The intervention should be replicated in other settings and, if it maintains effectiveness in different environments, should then be disseminated. In these latter stages, the central component is process evaluation, often using qualitative research methods, ensuring that the program is delivered across a community in ways likely to maintain effectiveness. Finally, as programs become institutionalised, population surveys can be used to track outcomes and system quality-control measures used across larger regions or national program rollout.

These evaluations may require different sets of information, to inform policy-makers of the real-world potential for innovative public health interventions. However, no single approach represents the 'best' evaluation design for all replication and dissemination purposes. One overarching principle is that in all evaluation studies, it is essential that the evaluation design and methods are well described. This includes an obligation to fully describe potential sources of bias, the sampling methods used and methods of data analysis in any report on an evaluation study. This is needed for all levels of intervention testing, replication (demonstration), dissemination and institutionalisation.

References

Borawski EA, Trapl ES, Adams-Tufts K et al. 2009, 'Taking Be Proud! Be Responsible! to the suburbs: a replication study', *Perspectives on Sexual and Reproductive Health*, vol. 41, no. 1, pp. 12–22.

Brownson RC, Colditz GA & Proctor EK (eds) 2012, *Dissemination and Implementation Research in Health: Translating Science to Practice*, Oxford University Press, New York, NY.

Dunton GF, Lagloire R & Robertson T 2009, 'Using the RE-AIM framework to evaluate the statewide dissemination of a school-based physical activity and nutrition curriculum: "Exercise Your Options"', *American Journal of Health Promotion*, vol. 23, no. 4, pp. 229–32.

Green LW & Glasgow RE 2006, 'Evaluating the relevance, generalization, and applicability of research: issues in external validation and translation methodology', *Evaluation and the Health Professions*, vol. 29, no. 1, pp. 126–53.

Green LW, Ottoson JM & Garcia C et al. 2009, 'Diffusion theory and knowledge dissemination, utilization, and integration in public health', *Annual Review of Public Health*, vol. 30, pp. 151–74.

Hooker SP, Seavey W & Weidmer CE et al. 2005, 'The California active aging community grant program: translating science into practice to promote physical activity in older adults', *Annals of Behavioral Medicine*, vol. 29, no. 3, pp. 155–65.

Layne JE, Sampson SE & Mallio CJ et al. 2008, 'Successful dissemination of a community-based strength training program for older adults by peer and professional leaders: the People Exercising Program', *Journal of the American Geriatrics Society*, vol. 56, no. 12, pp. 2323–9.

Manfredi C, Cho YI & Warnecke R et al. 2011, 'Dissemination strategies to improve implementation of the PHS smoking cessation guideline in MCH public health clinics: experimental evaluation results and contextual factors', *Health Education Research*, vol. 26, no. 2, pp. 348–60.

Milat AJ, King L & Bauman A et al. 2011, 'Scaling up health promotion interventions: an emerging concept in implementation science', *Health Promotion Journal of Australia*, vol. 22, no. 3, p. 238.

Rabin BA, Brownson RC & Haire-Joshu D et al. 2008, 'A glossary for dissemination and implementation research in health', *Journal of Public Health Management and Practice*, vol. 14, no. 2, pp. 117–23.

Reynolds KD, Buller DB & French SA et al. 2012, 'School sun-protection policies: measure development and assessments in 2 regions of the United States', *Journal of School Health*, vol. 82, no. 11, pp. 499–507.

Rychetnik L, Bauman A & Laws R et al. 2012, 'Translating research for evidence-based public health: key concepts and future directions', *Journal of Epidemiology and Community Health*, vol. 66, no. 12, pp. 1187–92.

Stewart AL, Grossman M & Bera N et al. 2006, 'Multilevel perspectives on diffusing a physical activity promotion program to reach diverse older adults', *Journal of Aging and Physical Activity*, vol. 14, no. 3, pp. 270–87.

Trickett EJ, Beehler S & Deutsch C et al. 2011, 'Advancing the science of community-level interventions', *American Journal of Public Health*, vol. 101, no. 8, pp. 1410–19.

Vidrine JI, Rabius V, Alford MH et al. 2010, 'Enhancing dissemination of smoking cessation quitlines through T2 translational research: a unique partnership to address disparities in the delivery of effective cessation treatment', *Journal of Public Health Management* and Practice, vol. 16, no. 4, pp. 304–8.

Wilson PM, Petticrew M & Calnan MW et al. 2010, 'Disseminating research findings: what should researchers do? A systematic scoping review of conceptual frameworks', *Implementation Science*, vol. 5, no. 91.

8

Evidence, practice, policy and the critical practitioner

The need to get research evidence into practice is partly determined by the policies, priorities and needs of decision-makers. This chapter summarises some of the issues that impede or facilitate research translation and use in the public health system. In addition, all practitioners need skills in critical appraisal of evidence, which are presented here, enabling good decisions to be made on the strength and usefulness of published evidence.

8.1 Getting evidence into practice

Improving the quality and effectiveness of health promotion interventions ultimately depends on our ability to use the evidence generated through research and evaluation. The central purpose of evaluation is to guide improvements in practice, through the application and adoption of interventions that have an impact on health and quality of life.

The use of evidence to guide decision-making in health promotion varies considerably and there are good reasons why this will be the case. In some circumstances sufficient 'evidence' of effectiveness does not exist and/or may be difficult to conclusively establish in a timely way. For example, when a new public health threat emerges (a communicable disease such as SARS), the need for rapid intervention demands a response in advance of good evidence from careful research. In other cases where new and complex public health problems (such as obesity) emerge, there may be considerable disagreement on the best mix of interventions to address the problem on a population basis (education, environmental change, regulation and so on). For policy-makers and practitioners, doing nothing in the absence of conclusive evidence is not an option.

On the other hand, adopting ineffective interventions is also unlikely to contribute to population health. In the absence of effectiveness or efficacy data, policy-makers sometimes have to prioritise the best available evidence on the basis of what works; this should be based on results from existing studies in the field and on information from practitioners and consumers (Glasgow et al. 2012). These programs should be be highly acceptable in practice, demonstrate the potential for high population reach, and always should be evaluated and assessed as they are implemented in a population, as an important part of public health expenditure and accountability.

Differences in the use of evidence in health promotion programs are indicated in Figure 8.1. One stage does not lead to another, but there is a proposed hierarchy that suggests superior practice will be based on the use of theory and research evidence.

The *planned* approach is exemplified by the use of planning models and logic models, as described in Chapters 1 and 2. This approach is based on rational, systematic assessment of the best available evidence concerning population health needs, effective interventions and the organisational and administrative conditions needed for successful intervention. This type of planning model represents evidence-based practice in health promotion, and links planning and evaluation in a logical sequence. Perceived community needs and the conditions necessary for the successful implementation of programs are accounted for in the planning process and through formative evaluation studies.

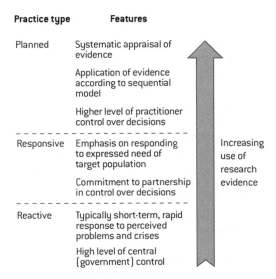

Figure 8.1 Variation in the use of evidence in health promotion: planned, responsive and reactive practice (adapted from Nutbeam 1996)

The *responsive* approach to health promotion reflects a common situation for practitioners and policy-makers. It is typified by many community programs that place high value on the role of a community in defining health priorities and participating in their solution. In this case the *response* is to the perceived needs of an identified population. This includes decisions about priorities and preferred forms of intervention, sometimes, but not always, informed by conventional 'evidence'. Such an orientation makes good sense as there is some evidence that communities involved in decisions about interventions are more likely to become involved in the intervention and to sustain its effects. But there are potential opportunity costs associated with responding to perceived community needs without sufficient consideration of the nature of the problems identified, or the evidence available about effective interventions.

Reactive practice is epitomised by short-term responses to a perceived problem, or real (or perceived) public health crisis. Typically, resources are made available through a government agency for an urgent and usually high-profile response. Often this practice does not allow for an evidence-based response, except possibly in the effective use of the mass media. Success might be seen in terms of a high level of message penetration, and in some cases the relief of political pressure to be seen to act. Examples include public education campaigns that promote abstinence in illicit drug use, or use fear to communicate risk in relation to HIV prevention. Evidence available from the evaluation of this type of campaign suggests that, although the campaign may improve knowledge of explicit risks and provide reassurance that 'something is being done', it may also have negative consequences, such as reinforcing existing prejudice about HIV infection and illicit drug misuse in the examples given. A more comprehensive approach, and hence complex program evaluation, may make a greater public health impact on these 'difficult' problems.

Health promotion practice includes a wide range of interventions that make use of theory and research in greatly varying ways. Although Figure 8.1 suggests a hierarchy of practice that places highest value on the use of traditional research evidence through a rational planning model, this is not always the preferred approach of practitioners, who may use a wider set of criteria to decide on priorities and intervention options. Practitioners who adopt a highly structured approach to program planning may find themselves in an uncomfortable position of being less able to respond to expressed community needs (a rewarding way to work) and political imperatives (a pragmatic way to work).

One of the frustrations facing diligent practitioners (and policy-makers) who want to use evidence to steer their decision-making is the paucity of relevant evaluation studies in the general literature on public health and health promotion. In reviewing the literature on any given topic, we typically find much research that describes the problem, but little intervention research that helps to identify practical population-level responses (Milat 2012). Further, many of the intervention studies reported in the literature are described as 'efficacious', but are often carried out in selected samples of people who participate in the research, or determine that interventions are efficacious, but only in smaller subgroups. Seldom do researchers highlight 'negative findings' or suggest that interventions should be discontinued, although this would be of considerable benefit to decision-makers.

Research on health inequalities provides a good example of this frustration. In looking for evidence from evaluated interventions to guide practice in tackling health inequalities, there is often an inverse relationship between the volume and quality of available research, and the potential effectiveness of the interventions researched. For example, the greater volume of evidence on potential interventions comes from studies designed to modify individual behavioural risks. This research has often been conducted with specially selected populations that are not representative of the social groups that need to be reached to reduce health inequalities, providing what some commentators have seen as the right answer to the wrong question. By contrast, there is little intervention research to assess the effectiveness of interventions to tackle some of the wider social, economic and environmental determinants of health. There is very little evidence of any kind to examine the relative costs and benefits of different intervention options.

It follows that research evidence can be used more effectively in practice if researchers, and those agencies that fund public health research, recognise the importance of conducting practice-relevant research. A great deal of practice-relevant evidence can be gathered instead from programs already in existence, by observing the way they operate, identifying what has worked in the past and what has not, and learning from the experience of practitioners in delivering programs. Some additional impact evaluation may be possible: for example, a pre–post research design to evaluate a community-wide obesity intervention may show that participants lose an average of four kilograms following an intensive dietary, policy and environmental intervention. This effect is likely to be due to the intervention, as people in communities without any intervention (the background state) lose no weight. This example illustrates the potential usefulness of non-randomised research designs in assessing effects in population-wide health promotion interventions.

Evidence gathered from investigations of these types is often presented in the form of case studies, reflecting expert opinion or even anecdotal evidence. Such 'evidence' generally ranks at the bottom of established hierarchies of evidence but both practitioners and policy-makers value it, particularly as it is often available when needed, and offers practical solutions that can be implemented.

In real-life circumstances, practitioners look to achieve the optimal balance between conventional evidence of efficacy and effectiveness, and the flexibility of response that is required at the heart of modern population-level practice. Unsurprisingly, in this book we advocate a planned approach to health promotion practice that makes fullest use of established theory and evidence of effectiveness, but we also recognise that in real-life circumstances, adaptations are often needed.

8.2 Getting evidence into policy

Many of the frustrations experienced by practitioners are similar for policy-makers. The role of evidence in public policy-making has been described and explained in widely varying ways. These range from a direct role for research in framing policy, and examples of evidence leading directly to policy change, through to evidence being considered an optional extra—a small part of a complex process in which evidence is used selectively to justify predetermined positions that are largely ideologically driven. Though there are obvious exceptions, neither extremity in this range is sustainable.

Most policy change is incremental and based on a mix of influences. When opportunities for policy reform open up, policy-makers will draw on available evidence, but policy change is often significantly constrained by established structures, investments and interests, and for these reasons is inherently political in nature. In this context, evidence is most often used if it fits with policy direction, and points to practical actions. Disappointingly, in health promotion we too frequently fail one or more of these tests.

Researchers are often surprised that the research they report in academic journals is ignored by policy-makers. Although most of us are committed to evidence-based policy-making, we tend to overlook the extent to which the choice of research, duration of funding, methods of communicating findings, and involvement in the policy process can interfere significantly with the achievement of this goal. Just like practitioners, policy-makers are keen to learn from existing programs, identifying what has worked in the past and learning from case studies. Such 'evidence' is valued by policy-makers, particularly as it is more likely to be available when needed, addresses issues of current concern, and offers solutions that are practical for implementation— the key conditions indicated above.

Regrettably, it is too often the case that the research questions of greatest interest to health promotion practitioners, and the policy-makers who make resources available, are not the questions that the researchers were funded to answer. As indicated above, too much research produces the right answers to the wrong questions. This means that decision-makers and practitioners can often be frustrated in finding program evaluation information that is really useful to them. Solutions to this impasse have to come from dialogue between researchers, practitioners and policy-makers to improve the relevance of the research done, and make the findings from research and evaluation studies as relevant to practice as possible.

The generation and deployment of research evidence for health promotion is an evolving field. Increasingly, the evaluations of health promotion programs are seen as multidisciplinary collaborations, with requirements for more timely and population-relevant outputs. What will also be obvious from the preceding chapters is that it is very risky to make decisions about the effectiveness of programs based on the results of a single study.

Much has been achieved in the development of methods for building, appraising and synthesising evidence, but bridging the 'gap' between this and the complexities of policy and practice remains a challenge. Part of the answer to this challenge comes from the differing approaches to 'translation research' (replication and dissemination) that are described in Chapter 7, testing promising ideas in different operating conditions and different places, and assessing how best to scale up a successful intervention. Replication and dissemination need to be carried out, tested and demonstrated, for the elements of effective programs suitable for population change to be identified.

> *Working out what components work and which can be translated across different settings and social groups are of greater importance to achieve population health gain.*

8.3 Critical appraisal of research and evaluation evidence

A major purpose of *Evaluation in a Nutshell* is to equip the reader with the ability to understand, interpret and assess the quality of published work in evaluation reports and in scientific journal papers. The preceding chapters have provided an introduction to many of the strategic and technical issues that arise in designing an evaluation, and some of the challenges in conducting program evaluations. Understanding the issues in program evaluation will help in making make judgments about the quality and relevance of 'evidence' that you may read in the published research literature.

This ability to 'critically appraise' the published evidence is an important skill for all practitioners, researchers and decision-makers. There is the appraisal of the 'science', and also of the policy and population relevance of the effects of a program. *Critical appraisal* in health promotion can be a complex process, requiring a broad approach to judging the worth of interventions; this may need a conscious trade-off between the quality of evidence (as assessed by scientific and methodological rigour) and the practicality for implementation (often a question of judgment on a program's applicability to local circumstances).

Appendix 6 provides a critical appraisal checklist through which the health promotion relevance as well as the methodological rigour of a published study can be appraised (Bauman & Rissel 2003). Building on the key messages from each of the previous chapters, the checklist clearly summarises the quality criteria for assessing formative, process and impact evaluation.

It is obvious that there is no single 'correct' answer for all forms of evaluation study. For example, in a local pilot program, emphasis might be placed on excellence in formative and process evaluation. For judging excellence in effectiveness and efficacy studies, the standard criteria for assessing 'scientific' quality are used—evaluation design, measurement, sample size, and appropriate approaches to the analyses of the results—but the relevance to local contexts, and potential for whole population reach, should also be considered.

This checklist could be used for reading any published evaluation in a peer-reviewed journal or monograph format. Starting with the problem definition, Part A of the checklist includes careful documentation of elements of formative and process evaluation (steps 2 and 3 in Appendix 6), as well as describing and assessing the quality of scientific research methods used. By the time the discussion of the published paper is reached, an attempt should be made to assess the practice-based relevance and generalisability of the findings, and whether the evaluation comprehensively covered all the components of good program evaluation.

Criteria for the searching for the later phases of evaluation are shown in Part B of the checklist (steps 6 to 8 in Appendix 6). For example, you might be searching for replication studies or evidence of successful dissemination of a project before considering the local adoption of a program. A search for replication studies may include the *grey literature*, which comprises less formal evaluations, published technical reports or monographs and other documents. Many of these evaluation reports from public sector or not-for-profit agencies are available through the internet. Though it is important to be cautious in assessing the scientific quality of information that does not come from peer-reviewed literature, these reports sometimes offer insight into the practical issues of implementation that are less often described in typical journal articles.

Finally, thinking beyond the checklist, we need guidelines for summarising the quality of different types of evidence reviews that are available for a defined content area. These summaries use systematic research techniques to compare and combine results from several interventions in a specific area, and answer specific questions on their average or usual effects. There are databases in which summaries are located, including the Cochrane Public Health Group, for assessing health promotion interventions (see Table 8.1). Examples of several 'centres of excellence' in summarising and reviewing evidence of health promotion effectiveness are shown in Table 8.1.

If outcomes are very similar or identical in measurement, and research designs are similar, then a quantitative pooled analysis can summarise the net effects of a particular kind of intervention; this is known as a *meta-analysis*. In health promotion this is rare across studies, so meta-analysis is less frequent than in clinical and biomedical research. Nonetheless, there are some health promotion examples of meta-analytical evidence, included in Table 8.1.

The ability to find evidence by accessing relevant reported research, and the ability to critically appraise evidence, are core skills in health promotion.

These skills provide the platform for planning the evaluation of a new intervention or applying evaluation methods to a new context or setting.

Table 8.1 Examples of systematic reviews of health promotion evidence

Centres/organisations specialising in reviews of prevention and health promotion program effectiveness	Examples of content areas covered
Cochrane Public Health Group (CPHG), formerly the Health Promotion and Public Health (HPPH) Field, Australia (www.cochrane.org/search/reviews and http://ph.cochrane.org/home)	Cochrane Collaboration does many systematic reviews (S/R) and meta-analyses of clinical and public health areas. Of relevance to health promotion, examples include: interventions to reduce sexually transmitted infections; S/R of internet and technology health promotion interventions; effectiveness of nutritional supplements; effects of handwashing and incident childhood disease.

Centres/organisations specialising in reviews of prevention and health promotion program effectiveness	Examples of content areas covered
Evidence for Policy and Practice Information and Co-ordinating Centre (EPPI-Centre), University of London, UK (http://eppi.ioe.ac.uk/cms)	S/R and economic evaluations. Examples include: peer-delivered interventions for young people; S/R of incentive schemes to encourage positive health; S/R of social/environmental interventions to reduce childhood obesity.
National Institute of Clinical Excellence (NICE), UK (http://www.nice.org.uk/#panel3)	Public health guidance. Clinical and public health sections; advice summaries described as 'guidance', practice focused. Examples include: economic evaluations of intensive home visiting programs for vulnerable families; S/R of participatory processes in health promotion (HP); S/R of HP schools; guidance on preventing harmful drinking (of alcohol).
The Community Guide, USA (www.thecommunityguide.org)	Guide to community preventive services, including S/R and evidence-based recommendations. S/R of preventive interventions and HP, many areas, including health equity; preventing violence (injuries); cardiovascular risk factor reduction; effective immunisation programs; mental illness prevention; reducing HIV risk in communities.
Health Evidence, Canada (www.healthevidence.org)	Evidence-informed decision making. Diverse reviews, including: S/R of mobile phone messaging for prevention; S/R to increase quality of life among people with dementia; S/R and meta-analysis of lifestyle interventions to prevent weight gain in young adults.

8.4   Concluding comments: evaluation—art and science

A major purpose of *Evaluation in a Nutshell* is to provide an introduction to technical issues in evaluation, and some of the challenges related to the evaluation of health promotion programs. What becomes clear from this introduction is that evaluating a health promotion intervention is both an art and a science.

The challenges we face stem from the diverse origins, goals and methods of health promotion programs. It should be clear throughout the book that evaluation should be integrated into a program plan from the beginning of a program idea (and the formative research that supports it), through to widespread program dissemination that should lead to population health change. Different evaluation designs and research methods are required for the different stages of program development, implementation and dissemination.

The various needs of researchers and practitioners often result in the use of a range of qualitative and quantitative methods, producing 'evidence' for different purposes. Given this diversity, we need to make decisions about the extent, expenditure and methodological rigour required for a particular program evaluation. We work in an imperfect environment and need to make the method fit the circumstances of the intervention. There is no single, correct evaluation design. Both qualitative and quantitative methods have an important place; both can be done well and both done badly, and one is not superior to the other.

For every health promotion intervention, careful formative and process evaluations are essential. Good program development and clear planning will ensure that a quality program is developed; careful monitoring of implementation will contribute to an understanding of why one program works and another does not. Process evaluation is often neglected, but contributes to an understanding of the way the program worked that can inform subsequent program development and refinement. Process evaluation provides the foundation for subsequent evaluation of program effectiveness, and is the cornerstone of the evaluation of replication and dissemination of programs.

To evaluate the effectiveness of a program, especially when a program is being implemented for the first time, randomised controlled or quasi-experimental designs are the minimum standards for evaluation design. Established, reliable and valid impact measures should be used. The results should be assessed in terms of the observed *effect size*. Both qualitative and quantitative methods have an important place and, together, they can provide different perspectives. This combination of perspectives can provide information on the acceptability and feasibility of interventions, as well as providing evidence of effectiveness.

Effective interventions need to be replicated in different settings to assess if they can be conducted and delivered to diverse populations. If replication shows the program is possible in other settings, then policy-makers and practitioners need to be influenced to adopt and disseminate the program more widely. Only when an effective program is delivered across a whole region in a sustainable way can it produce population-level health benefit.

Ultimately, not all of us have the opportunity or resources to undertake highly structured evaluation of our work. Better knowledge of the strategic and technical issues in health promotion evaluation not only enables us make well-informed judgments of published work but also enables us to better judge when, how and to what level we may need to evaluate our own work as *critical practitioners*. This knowledge is also of great importance in managing the expectations of managers, funders and the wider community.

References

Bauman A & Rissel C 2003, 'Guidelines for journal reviewing', *Health Promotion Journal of Australia*, vol. 4, no. 2, pp. 79–82.

Glasgow RE, Green LW & Taylor MV et al. 2012, 'An evidence integration triangle for aligning science with policy and practice', *American Journal of Preventive Medicine*, vol. 42, no. 6, pp. 646–54.

Milat AJ, Bauman AE & Redman S et al. 2011, 'Public health research outputs from efficacy to dissemination: a bibliometric analysis', *BMC Public Health*, vol. 11.

Nutbeam, D 1996, 'Achieving "best practice" in health promotion: improving the fit between research and practice', *Health Education Research*, vol. 11, no. 3, pp. 317–26.

appendices

Appendix 1 CONSORT criteria for randomised trials

These criteria are used for randomised trials; compare them with the TREND criteria in Appendix 5, which are the criteria for non-randomised studies. Many scientific journals use this checklist to support standardisation of reporting on controlled trials.

Among the key elements included in the CONSORT checklist are:

- definition of clear eligibility criteria (who is included in the study) and recruitment;
- random allocation of the participants to intervention and control groups;
- measurement of the characteristics of the study sample (intervention and control groups) before the intervention is implemented (age, gender, ethnicity, social background and so on);
- use of a sufficient number of participants in both intervention and control groups (*sample size*) to detect expected effects;
- full description of the intervention and assessment of its implementation (process evaluation);
- identical assessment, applied to people after the intervention using *reliable* and *valid* measures (ensuring that all subjects are assessed regardless of exposure to the intervention);
- analysis of the observed differences between intervention and non-intervention groups using appropriate statistical techniques;
- discussion of the *representativeness* of the study group of the population from which it was sampled.

CONSORT Statement for Reporting Randomised Trials, www.consort-statement.org, is recommended for further reading.

Appendix 2 Statistical tests and methods: a hypothetical intervention to prevent diabetes

Imagine that a hypothetical weight-loss intervention targeting people at high risk of developing diabetes was delivered to 100 people, using 100 controls with a randomised controlled design. Assume that:

- very careful measurement (assessment) was made of participants' weight, using reliable and valid measuring scales;
- excellent follow-up was possible;
- participants were weighed 12 months later to assess the impact of the intervention on their weight;
- participants were also assessed five years later to assess the outcome of developing diabetes, identifying all new cases of diabetes (this is good measurement);
- all 100 participants had baseline and end-of-program weight data;
- all participants had five-year follow-up data on whether or not they had developed diabetes.

The *impact* assessment (short-term to intermediate outcome) here is of a continuously measured variable (weight in kilograms), and the five-year *outcome* is categorical (whether or not participants developed diabetes). Simple statistical methods for analysing these data are shown, and the purpose of Table A2.1 is to show analyses for continuous data (weight in kilograms), and categorical data (outcome of developing diabetes or not).

Table A2.1 Examples of statistical techniques and analysis in a hypothetical (and effective) weight-loss intervention

Weight-loss intervention					
Groups (1 group = 100 people)	Baseline average weight (kg)[1] (SD)	12-month follow-up average weight (kg) (SD)	Difference in weight (SD)[2]	Statistical test and p value[3]	95% confidence intervals for the difference[4]
Intervention n = 100 adults	91.15 kg (4.76)	86.40 kg (5.30)	4.75 kg	t-test within intervention group, t = 28.6, p < 0.001	4.42 to 5.07 kg
Control n = 100 adults	91.35 kg (4.69)	91.23 kg (5.73)	0.12 kg	t-test within control group, t = 0, 7m, p = 0.52	−0.25 to 0.49 kg

(*continued*)

Table A2.1 *continued*

Weight-loss intervention					
Groups (1 group = 100 people)	Baseline average weight (kg)[1] (SD)	12-month follow-up average weight (kg) (SD)	Difference in weight (SD)[2]	Statistical test and p value[3]	95% confidence intervals for the difference[4]
Between group statistical comparison			4.63 kg	t-test of the difference between groups, t = 18.6, p < 0.001	4.13 to 5.12 kg
Development of diabetes at five-year follow-up					
Categorical data (n = 100 people in each group)	Percentage free from diabetes at baseline	Percentage free from diabetes	New cases of diabetes (incidence)[5]	Relative risk (RR) of developing diabetes[6]	
Intervention	n = 100 (100%)	n = 90 (90%)	n = 10 (10%)	RR = 0.33[7]	0.17 to 0.64
Control	n = 100 (100%)	n = 70 (70%)	n = 30 (30%)		

The hypothetical data set used in this example is available online for your own analysis at www.mhhe.com/au/bauman2e.

1 Weight is a *continuous* measure, and the average (mean) weight is 91.3 kilograms in this sample.

2 SD = standard deviation, a measure of the variation around the measured weight in this sample.

3 The p values show the probability of this size of weight loss occurring by chance; for the intervention group, the weight loss of 4.75 kilograms is unlikely to have happened by chance (very small p value); for the control group, the weight loss of only 0.12 kilograms is not significant (i.e. not a real weight loss). Note that the difference between groups, 4.63 kilograms, shows a very small p value, unlikely to be by chance. So, this is described as a significant difference in weight loss between groups.

4 These confidence intervals describe a range of values within which the true value is likely to lie (in the underlying target population). The 95 per cent confidence intervals show that in the intervention group, the likely range of weight loss in the underlying target population is between 4.42 and 5.07 kilograms and, for the controls, between a weight *gain* of 0.25 kilograms, and a weight *loss* of 0.49 kilograms. For other writings on 95 per cent confidence intervals, consult the further reading list.

5 Incidence of diabetes: the number of new cases of diabetes developing over five years (this is a *categorical* measure).

6 Relative risk (RR): the rate of those remaining obese in the intervention group, compared to the rate in the control group.

7 This shows that the rate of developing diabetes in the intervention group is one-third of that seen in controls (RR 0.33), and that the confidence intervals suggest the true relative risk lies somewhere in the range between one in six (= 0.17), and nearly two-thirds (= 0.64).

Additional analyses were carried out. These analyses are beyond the scope of this book, but illustrate an important idea: irrespective of group, those who lost three or more kilograms were less likely to develop diabetes (only four out of 98 developed diabetes) than those who lost only one or two kilograms or who gained weight (36 out of 102 developed diabetes). The latter group were eight times more likely to develop diabetes than those who lost weight. This is an example of a *mediator*, weight loss. The intervention led to weight loss, which in turn led to reduced diabetes risk.

Intervention ⟹ Weight loss ⟹ Diabetes

The data set for these analyses is available online at www.mhhe.com/au/bauman2e.

Appendix 3 Examples of techniques and methods commonly used to assess measurement reliability and validity

Table A3.1 Some examples of techniques and methods used to assess measurement reliability and validity

Type of reliability or validity	Typical statistical methods used	Example from a health promotion measurement study: purpose of the measurement development	Examples of the statistics and coefficients used for measurement development purposes in the study
Reliability			
Test–re-test repeatability	Usually *intra-class correlation* (ICC); sometimes *Spearman's rho* for non-parametric data (skewed distributions)	Wiens et al. (2010) tested a Canadian adaptation of the SmartDiet questionnaire in assessing fat and fibre intake.	Test–re-test repeatability as shown for fat and fibre intake (ICC values 0.66 and 0.74 respectively), indicating stability of dietary habits in this sample.[1]
	For categorical data (data in two or a few categories) *kappa* coefficient is often used.	Test–re-test repeatability was ascertained by administering the same questions one month apart.	

(*continued*)

Table A3.1 *continued*

Type of reliability or validity	Typical statistical methods used	Example from a health promotion measurement study: purpose of the measurement development	Examples of the statistics and coefficients used for measurement development purposes in the study
Reliability			
Inter-rater reliability	Assessing two raters to measure agreement (usually, *ICC* or *kappa* coefficient are used).	Berkson et al. (2012) examined agreement in assessing height and weight of school students by physical education teachers in the USA.	Excellent agreement between raters, with ICC values > 0.95 in controlled and field settings; < 2% discrepant values noted; suggests teachers can be trained to accurately measure height and weight of children; potentially useful in obesity surveillance.
Responsiveness	This tests a measure's capacity to respond in an effective program: usual analytic methods are used to assess statistical significance, such as a t-test (if continuous data) or an odds ratio (if categorical).	This is identical to measuring change following a program; outcome needs to show measurable change in response to an effective intervention; a responsive measure shows significant changes in intervention groups and limited change in controls (see Chapter 5, Figure 5.1).	Standard tests for significance of observed differences: all usual statistical tests might be used to demonstrate responsiveness (t-tests, non-parametric tests, chi-squared tests, odds ratios with 95% confidence intervals). For example, Krebs (2010) showed responsiveness of different self-report pain measures following an intervention.
Validity			
Criterion validity	Compares a new measure to an established 'true', objective measure of the factor of interest; uses various psychometric or epidemiological coefficients.	Taylor et al. (2011): rated the quality of parks for physical activity, auditing 50 randomly chosen urban parks, using Google Earth.	Comparing Google Earth scores with an established directly observed measure of parks, the POST score. Correlation of 0.9 overall, and good association with most park dimensions.

Type of reliability or validity	Typical statistical methods used	Example from a health promotion measurement study: purpose of the measurement development	Examples of the statistics and coefficients used for measurement development purposes in the study
Validity			
Construct validity	Whether the score or scale measures an underlying non-observed theoretical construct; usually demonstrated techniques, such as *factor analysis*.	Gouveia (2009) assessed a 'satisfaction with life' measure in 2180 Brazilians from different population samples to assess if there was one underlying 'score' or construct.	Confirmatory factor analysis showed that there was one underlying construct measuring 'life satisfaction' (so, it could be treated as one score). All questions (items) were important (related to overall score, with very good Cronbach alpha coefficients ~ 0.8).

1 In addition, criterion validity was assessed in this study by comparing the self-report questionnaires against an objective measure, a three-day food record (a validation study).

Appendix 4 Economic evaluations in a nutshell

Several levels of economic evaluation are relevant to health promotion programs, especially to complex programs, as there are multiple components (inputs or expenditures) to be considered in relation to outcomes.

First, in a program of work or area of work, assess the overall relative expenditure on health promotion and disease prevention, relative to overall health expenditure. Taking a broader 'health in all' policy approach, the costs of a complex health promotion program may need to be considered within other budgets as well (transport, urban planning, agriculture, education, sport crime/justice, as well as the health budget).

Next is simple costing of health promotion programs. What does a project or overall program cost? What is the cost per unit change in an outcome? (For example, what is the cost per smoker who quits, or cost per kilogram of weight loss, calculated simply as 'kg lost/total project costs'?). Economists are interested in approaches very relevant to health promotion, for example, efficiency (maximises the benefit for given resources); technical efficiency (can resources be spent in alternate ways to produce the same output from a health promotion program?); allocative efficiency (equity focus; is the right mix of programs being delivered?).

Finally, economic analyses in health promotion are most often cost-effectiveness studies (costs/unit change in outcome), cost–utility analysis (costs/QALY or DALY, so that programs can be compared), and cost–benefit analysis (where outcomes are monetised).

Appendix 5 TREND statement (Transparent Reporting of Evaluation with Non-randomised Designs)

This TREND statement provides a 22-item checklist for non-randomised trials, with a focus relevant for CPE (Des Jarlais et al. 2004). It orients researchers towards external validity (generalisability), rather than only focusing on internal validity. The checklist includes items concerning:

- the target population: whom is the intervention or program trying to influence?
- the underpinning theory/framework (for behaviour change);
- eligibility/inclusion of participants: how are they sampled?; what are the settings for recruitment?
- sample size chosen (power), approaches to analysis;
- how participants are allocated to the intervention group(s);
- choice of measures: what impact/outcome factors are chosen?
- units of analysis: whether individual or group change is sought;
- participant flow through the study: how people are engaged in the intervention after recruitment;
- baseline equivalence: whether intervention and comparison groups of people are similar before the intervention;
- interpretation of results: how results are considered in terms of their generalisability.

Appendix 6 Critical appraisal checklist for health promotion programs

This appendix has been adapted and updated from Bauman A & Rissel C 2003, 'Guidelines for journal reviewing', *Health Promotion Journal* of *Australia*, vol. 4, no. 2, pp. 79–82.

Part A: the appraisal of individual interventions

1. **Problem definition**
   - Is the health problem a health promotion priority?
   - What is the magnitude of the problem, and which population subgroups are at risk?

2. **Formative evaluation and program development**
   - Is the problem amenable to change, through a feasible intervention (check the literature)? Are interventions published in this area and were they effective? If there are several studies in the literature, are there summaries of the evidence in this area (non-systematic or selective reviews; planned systematic reviews; or formal pooled estimates from multiple studies (using statistical techniques of meta-analysis)?
   - Is there evidence of piloting or testing of the intervention or its component parts?
   - Was the intervention tested with people similar to the proposed target group?
   - Is there an underlying theoretical framework or conceptual model for the intervention?
   - Are the intervention strategies and settings identified as 'best practice' approaches?
   - Are there funds for the intervention to be delivered as planned, and is there sufficient time for expected effects or changes to be observed?
   - Is there a logic model to describe the ways that the intervention/program might work?

3. **Process evaluation**
   - Is there evidence of process evaluation to monitor the implementation of the program components?
   - Is there evidence that the program was well-received by the target population?
   - Is there evidence of adaptation of the intervention, fitting the intervention into different settings (and whether the effects of the program were similar in different contexts)?
   - How many people received (attended, participated in) the intervention? Were they typical of the target group at large (or: were they different to those who did not participate)? Of all those who could participate or be included, how many actually did so?

4. **Research methods to appraise the stages of impact and outcome evaluation**

Study (research) design

■ What was the study (research) design in this evaluation? Was it the most feasible study design that might have been used in this setting within available resources? Will the design provide sufficient evidence of effectiveness?

Study sample

■ What is the target population? Are the people who actually participated in the intervention typical of the target population?

■ How were people recruited into, or how did they volunteer for, the study?

■ What were the *selection effects* that might influence (bias) this study (e.g. non-representative volunteer samples used in the studies that generated the evidence)?

Measurement

■ Are there specified and measurable intervention objectives?

■ Are all relevant outcomes assessed? How important are any omitted outcomes?

■ Were the measuring tools, questionnaire or instruments reliable and valid?

Analysis

■ Was the sample size of participants in the study (or those measured)—i.e. the statistical power of the study—sufficient to detect any potential effects that might result from the intervention?

■ Were there any factors that were not measured that might have influenced the findings?

■ Were any of these extraneous influencing factors controlled for in the statistical analysis?

■ Were the most appropriate approaches to analyses used?

General

■ Is the time frame for the proposed change clearly stated? Is it realistic?

■ Is there other corroborating evidence of the observed effects (either from changes in other outcomes or from qualitative evaluation data)?

■ (Specifically for complex program evaluations (CPEs)). Is there evidence of an integrated set of planning tasks, and organised program implementation? Were all components evaluated using appropriate methods (quantitative and qualitative)? Is there corroborative evidence from the evaluation of multiple interlinked program components?

5. **Interpretation/discussion of the results**
   - Were the conclusions drawn by the author(s) justified by their data?
   - Were the findings generalisable to the whole community or to similar populations/settings?
   - Were any reported significant effects of actual practical health promotion significance or were they simply of statistical significance?
   - Did the formative or process evaluation components of the evaluation enable us to understand how or why the the health promotion program worked? Especially for negative studies, might additional information have been informative here?
   - Is there a need for replication research in this area or, if the intervention appeared to be ineffective, what other approaches might be developed to address this problem?

Part B: post-intervention appraisal—making a public health difference?

6. **Replication**
   - Has the initial effective/efficacious intervention subsequently been implemented and tested in a diverse range of settings?
   - Were these settings diverse enough to indicate the population generalisability of this intervention?
   - Were the programs implemented and delivered successfully (mostly adhering to program objectives and methods) in these different settings; or, if implementation differed, what difference did adaptation make to outcomes observed?
   - Were the results communicated to policy-makers and to professionals and practitioners? Is there a defined advocacy strategy to communicate these results? (This is knowledge translation—see Rychetnik et al. 2012.)

7. **Dissemination**
   - What mechanisms for dissemination are suggested? What might be possible?
   - Is there evidence of policy-maker support and resources to assist dissemination?
   - What is the extent of efforts at dissemination and is it sufficient for *population reach*?

8. **Institutionalisation**

■ Are there policy changes in place to support and resource the institutionalisation of the effective and disseminated program?

■ Are there monitoring systems in place to assess program sustainability and quality control of the intervention/program (process evaluation)?

■ Are there surveillance systems to monitor the impact/outcomes of interest at the population level (e.g. rates of smoking in pregnancy, immunisation rates in pre-schoolers, new HIV-positive seroconversions per year)?

References

Berkson SS, Espinola J & Corso KA et al. 2013, 'Reliability of height and weight measurements collected by physical education teachers for a school-based body mass index surveillance and screening system', *Journal of School Health*, vol. 83, pp. 21–7.

Des Jarlais DC, Lyles C & Crepaz N et al. 2004, 'Improving the reporting quality of nonrandomized evaluations of behavioral and public health interventions: The TREND statement', *American Journal of Public Health*, vol. 94, no. 3, pp. 361–6.

Gouveia VV, Milfont TL & da Fonseca P et al. 2009, 'Life satisfaction in Brazil: testing the psychometric properties of the Satisfaction With Life Scale (SWLS) in five Brazilian samples', *Social Indicators Research*, vol. 90, pp. 267–77.

Krebs EE, Blair MJ & Damush T et al. 2010, 'Comparative responsiveness of pain outcome measures among primary care patients with musculoskeletal pain', *Medical Care*, vol. 48, pp. 1007–14.

Rychetnik L, Bauman A & Laws R et al. 2012, 'Translating research for evidence-based public health: key concepts and future directions', *Journal of Epidemiology and Community Health*, vol. 66, no. 12, pp. 1187–92.

Taylor BT, Fernando P & Bauman AE et al. 2011, 'Measuring the quality of public open space using Google Earth', *American Journal of Preventive Medicine*, vol. 40, no. 2, pp. 105–12.

Wiens L, Schulzer M & Chen C et al. 2010, 'Reliability and validity of the Smart Diet Canadian version questionnaire', *Journal of the American Dietetic Association*, vol. 110, no. 1, pp. 101–5.

glossary

Advocacy the combination of actions designed to gain policy support, political commitment, and professional and community acceptance for a particular course of action to promote or enhance health

Behavioural epidemiology the study of the distribution (how much of a problem in the population) and determinants of (causal factors that lead to) behaviours that are related to health. It contributes to an understanding of the individual, social and environmental factors and conditions that lead to health-enhancing or health-comprising behaviours. It overlaps with a *social epidemiology perspective*, which takes a 'social determinants' perspective on factors leading to health

Bias where something differs systematically from the true situation. Biases found in studies may be due to how people are selected or chosen or volunteer for a program (*selection bias*), how they are assessed or measured (*measurement or information bias*), or other factors that may influence the observations made or associations found through analysis of data (such as **confounding factors**)

Cluster randomised controlled trial a randomised controlled trial (RCT) where randomisation occurs at the level of groups or communities. These groups or communities are randomly allocated to intervention or control (comparison) conditions. This is necessary and appropriate where individuals within a community share features in common (are clustered), such as in work sites or school classes. See also **randomised controlled trial (RCT)**

Cohort an identified group or population. In a cohort study, the same population is followed and assessed at each stage in the study, both before and after an intervention. Cohorts are sometimes used in **quasi-experimental design** studies

Complex program evaluation (CPE) the process of designing and conducting evaluations of complex (public health) programs; these are multi-component interventions targeting multi-faceted problems in whole populations or community settings, and using a range of diverse strategies to influence any or all of: individuals, settings, professionals or policy-makers

Concept an organising idea, often theoretical, used to describe a phenomenon that is not directly observable. In health promotion, we use concepts such as community capacity, self-efficacy and social influence, and then try to develop operational measures of them. See also **observable phenomena**

Confidence intervals a statistical term used to describe the extent to which the true results are outside of a range

The definitions in this glossary are pragmatic definitions based on the authors' experiences in evaluation, research and practice in health promotion. More formal definitions can be found in publications such as Last, JM 2000, *A Dictionary of Epidemiology*, Oxford University Press, Oxford, and Nutbeam, D 1999, 'Health promotion glossary', *Health Promotion International*, vol. 13, no. 4, pp. 349–64. A more recent update is Smith BJ, Tang KC & Nutbeam D 2006, 'WHO health promotion glossary: new terms', *Health Promotion International*, vol. 21, pp. 340–5.

of possible results described by the *confidence limits* (the confidence limits or confidence interval include a range of values within which the true value in the population is likely to lie). Note this is slightly different to *p-value*, which is an estimate of the probability of rejecting the null hypothesis of a study question (that the intervention did not work) when that hypothesis is true; in simple terms, a p-value describes whether effects are significant or not. The p-value is calculated using *parametric statistics*, based usually on an underlying normal distribution of data (see Appendix 2 for examples, such as the use of t-tests)

Confounding factors (confounders) variables that may influence the association between two other variables and thereby confound the results in a study. For example, a study may find that women have better preventive practices than men, indicating that gender is associated with preventive practices. However, another variable, not gender, may be causing this association. For example, women may have higher self-efficacy than men, and self-efficacy might be associated with preventive practices. Thus the relationship between gender and preventive practice may be due to differences in self-efficacy and not really due to gender itself. Here, self-efficacy is the confounder for the relationship between gender and preventive practice

Construct validity see **validity**

Consultation the process of engaging with or seeking the views of stakeholders or the community or target group members, with a view to enabling participation in intervention development, advocacy or policy formulation. See also **participatory planning**

Contamination the amount to which control or comparison groups or

communities might be exposed to intervention elements. For example, in a community-wide campaign, the control communities may share some media channels in common with intervention communities. If they are exposed to the campaign messages, it will be more difficult to show that program effects are greater in the intervention community than the control community

Content validity see **validity**

Correlates factors associated with other variables. For example, in a survey of teenagers, boys are more likely to be physically active than girls. It simply means that there is a statistical relationship between gender and physical activity. Correlation does not imply causality. See also **confounding factors** and **determinants**

Cross-sectional study a survey, or other form of data collection, that is obtained at a single point in time from a population or population sample. Unlike in a **cohort** study, these individuals are not followed and assessed on a further occasion

Determinants variables that 'cause' observed or measured outcomes. For example, cigarette smoking 'causes' lung cancer through a series of steps that have established a clear and unequivocal relationship between smoking behaviour and subsequent risk of lung cancer. Establishing similar, unequivocal relationships between health promotion outcomes (such as knowledge or social attitudes) and subsequent behaviours is a continuing area of research endeavour. We often misuse the term 'determinants' when we really mean that there is a **cross-sectional** statistical association between variables or that they are **correlates**

Dissemination an active and intentional process of achieving the maximum uptake of effective and feasible health promotion interventions into a community; a stage in research and evaluation where a program or intervention is scaled-up to reach a large population or population group

Drop out or loss to follow-up the proportion of participants who start a program or are included in a study, and do not participate in follow-up activities or surveys—they are 'lost to follow-up'. This may lead to **bias** in the results if those individuals who are followed up are systematically different from those not followed up. See also **non-response bias**

Effect size a quantitative metric that describes the size of the difference in **effectiveness** between intervention and control groups (in a standardised way that can be compared among studies)

Effectiveness the extent to which an intervention or program is successful in 'real-life' conditions in achieving the impact and outcomes that were predicted during the planning of the program

Efficacy the extent to which a health promotion intervention is successful (in achieving its proposed outcomes) under controlled or 'best possible' conditions; usually characterised by optimal scientific design

Evaluation the process of judging the value of something. In health promotion, an evaluation will determine the extent to which a program has achieved its desired outcomes, and will assess the different processes that led to these outcomes. Scientists, health practitioners, politicians and the wider community all have different views on what represents value from a health promotion program, how success should be defined and what

should be measured. Hence, there is no 'correct approach' to health promotion evaluation; it is context-specific. See also **formative evaluation, impact evaluation** and **process evaluation**

Evaluation design the set of procedures and tasks that need to be carried out to examine the effects of a health promotion intervention. The purpose of a good evaluation design is to enable us to be as confident as possible that the health promotion intervention caused any changes that were observed. This is similar to the terms *research design* or *study design*, which usually refer to the designs of the quantitative evaluation of program **effectiveness** or **efficacy**

Face validity see **validity**

Fidelity (also known as *program fidelity*) is part of **process evaluation** which examines whether or not the intervention/program was delivered using the methods and materials as designed and used as intended with the proposed target audiences

Formative evaluation a set of activities designed to develop, identify and test program materials and methods. Formative evaluation occurs as part of program planning, and occurs before any elements of the program are implemented

Generalisability the extent to which the findings from the study are likely to be reproduced in other groups or in the whole population. This is sometimes described as *external validity*. This contrasts with the degree to which the results are scientifically supported by the study itself—this is referred to as the *internal validity* of the results and describes how well the intervention was likely to *cause* the outcomes observed

Goals general statements describing the overall purpose and direction or the end-point outcomes being sought from an intervention or program; comprised of specific measurable **objectives**

Health literacy the capacity that individuals have or develop to locate and use information for improving conditions related to their health, improving their health or accessing needed services

Health outcomes the long-term end-points of a health promotion program. They may include reduced morbidity and mortality, improved quality of life and functional independence

Health promotion outcomes modifiable personal, social and environmental factors that are a means to changing the determinants of health (**intermediate health outcomes**). They also represent the more immediate results of planned health promotion activities

Impact evaluation a set of activities designed to assess short-term effects or **efficacy** of an intervention. This may include measurement of **intermediate health outcomes**

Indicators see **measures and indicators**

Institutionalisation where a program has been successfully diffused into a community, has established policy support and funding mechanisms, and has continuing community support. At this last stage, the program is integrated into the long-term functions of a host agency or organisation. This stage of evaluation is primarily concerned with quality control and long-term monitoring and surveillance of outcomes at a population level

Intermediate health outcomes the results of health promotion programs in the short term, which are measured by changes in lifestyle factors (for example, food choices, physical activity and substance use), accessing preventive services, or environment changes that are likely to lead to improved health outcomes

Internal consistency assesses how well a group of items or questions 'hang together'. It assesses the consistency of results across items within a score or scale. It describes how well each question relates independently to the rest of the questions in a scale and how they relate overall

Intervention see **project or intervention**

Logic model a way of describing the changes that the program is intended to bring about, defining what will happen during a program, in what order, and with what anticipated effects. This is a conceptual 'roadmap' or illustration of how the program elements might work. It is designed in the planning stages, and reflects how a program will be planned, implemented and with what proposed effects. It is a drawing or map that describes program inputs (human, financial and material resources), the context of the program (factors that will influence the implementation and impact of the intervention) and describes the activities that make up the intervention (such as program events, groups, training and social marketing). In turn, these are linked to the levels of outcomes that these 'inputs' are likely to produce. A logic model is similar to *intervention mapping*

Measures and indicators both assess and measure phenomena, but measures are usually related to impact and outcome evaluation, and are central to demonstrating **efficacy** or **effectiveness** of programs; they usually require demonstrated reliability and validity, as discussed in Chapter 5. There are a range of definitions for indicators, but these are often process evaluation measures, such as counts of phenomena, quality measures, measures of services, measures of policy or environments, or measures of **health promotion outcomes**

Meta-analysis the research process of quantitative pooling of effects from different interventions to obtain an average effect of the **effectiveness** across studies. It is an extension of a systematic review, which is a literature-review focused appraisal and synthesis of research evidence relevant to the effectiveness of a particular intervention or program (non-quantitative review)

Non-observable phenomena attributes or characteristics (such as knowledge, attitudes, public opinion, and even some health behaviours) that cannot be directly observed and measured, and have to be indirectly assessed (for example, through surveys that are self-completed or through questions asked in face-to-face or telephone interviews). See also **observable phenomena**

Non-response bias the differences in the variables of interest in a study between those participating in or completing a study (or intervention program) and those who **drop out** or do not participate. The term 'subject retention' is a related idea; it refers to the difference in the number of participants who start a program and those who actually complete it

Objectives health promotion program objectives are measurable changes to modifiable personal attributes (such as knowledge, motivations and skills), social norms and social support, and organisational factors (such as rules and processes) that influence the program goals. See also **health promotion outcomes**

Observable phenomena attributes or characteristics to be measured that are directly observable. For example, height and weight, blood pressure or

serum cholesterol levels can be assessed through direct measurement. See also **non-observable phenomena**

Outcome evaluation a set of activities designed to assess whether or not the program successfully achieved its *end-point goals* (such as changes in health behaviours) and *intermediate objectives* (such as improved knowledge and skills). Usually outcomes imply longer term changes such as health status, whereas shorter term end-points are often described as program impact. See also **impact evaluation**

Participatory planning a process of engaging with communities or stakeholders to form partnerships to plan and deliver programs. The program planning works with community participation to make shared decisions about the content and format of programs, or about changes that will impact on the community to improve health

Pilot testing a set of activities designed to assess the feasibility and/or relevance of intervention components (see **formative evaluation**). Pilot testing may also refer to measurement development and piloting of a measurement in a sample of people. This is used to assess the **reliability** and **validity** of the proposed measurement

Pre–post study a one group evaluation design (also known as a 'before–after study'). This is in the category of pre-experimental or non-experimental study designs. This is a relatively weak design, with one group or population measured before and after an intervention. This design is often used in pilot studies to estimate the likely effect of an intervention, and is not usually recommended for use in the detailed evaluation of innovative health promotion interventions

Prevalence a measure that describes how many people are affected by, or have, a particular problem in a defined population

Process evaluation a set of activities designed to assess the success and factors surrounding program implementation. Process evaluation describes and explains what happens once the program has actually started, and the extent to which the program is implemented and delivered as planned. See also **fidelity**

Program of work see **project or intervention**

Program plan usually a written document that specifies the interventions to be employed, the sequence of activities, the partnerships to be developed, the personnel to be involved at different stages and the costs of the interventions. See also **logic model**

Project or intervention compared to a program of work, a discrete project or intervention is usually based on the use of a single method or single intervention strategy in a clearly defined setting; a more comprehensive program of work, using multiple intervention/ project strategies in different settings and targeting multiple groups, requires more **complex program evaluation**

Qualitative methods descriptive and analytical research techniques that are used to explore and explain phenomena of interest. Methods include the use of focus groups (structured discussions with stakeholders or members of a target group) or directly learning from participating in or with target group members (ethnographic research or participant observation, sometimes called 'action research')

Quantitative methods descriptive and analytic research techniques that are intended to produce numeric data amenable to statistical analysis.

Such data allow statistical testing of comparisons between groups, trends over time or the strength of associations between variables

Quasi-experimental designs evaluation designs that have defined control or comparison populations against which intervention group effects could be compared. The population or group receiving the intervention is predetermined and non-randomly assigned. A pre–post design may be classified as a quasi-experimental design if there are multiple time points of observation. (For an example of a one group time series, see Chapter 5, Figure 5.2, example 5)

Random sample a **sample** drawn from a population where each individual has an equal probability of being chosen. Random sampling is intended to produce a sample of individuals that is representative of the population

Randomised controlled trial (RCT) a research design where the individuals (or groups) receiving the intervention are not predetermined. Individuals or groups are randomly allocated to receive the program (*intervention* or *experimental* group), or not to receive the program (*control* or *comparison* group). Every individual or group has an equal chance of being offered the program or not

Reach a term used to describe the proportion of a target population that is engaged in the elements of an intervention or program. Reach is important in determining the generalisability of a program to a population as a whole. The concept of reach is also relevant to the **replication** and **dissemination** stages of program evaluation. See also **generalisability**

Reliability the stability of a measure, assessing the extent to which, each time the measure is used and for each person it is used with, it will measure the same thing (give the same score or value). This is also referred to as 'test–re-test reliability'. Another form of assessment of reliability is *inter-rater reliability*, which is where two individuals assess the same phenomenon and the level of agreement between them is described

Replication the process of repeating an intervention in a different setting or with a different population or subgroup to assess whether intervention effects are similar or different

Representativeness usually of data or information from a sample of people, sample representativeness is important in program evaluation as it describes how well the observed data reflect the true data in the underlying population of people (from which the sample was drawn). If the results of an evaluation are from a representative sample, then the results will be more **generalisable**. If the sample is *randomly drawn* from a population, and of sufficient **sample size**, results are likely to be more representative

Responsiveness the capacity of a measurement for change in response to an intervention. The best responsive measures should show a substantial change following an intervention, but not show change in the absence of an intervention

Sample a group of individuals selected from a population for study, or to be the subjects for a health promotion intervention. See also **random sample**. Special types of samples are *convenient sampling* (non-probability samples, not randomly sampled, such as intercept surveys, or surveys of volunteers) and *snowball sampling* (these are also non-random or convenient samples, with people identified from a hard-to-reach target group, then finding other people like them; this snowball process results

in a substantial number of people from whom information can be collected)

Sample size is calculated by working out how many people are needed for an evaluation study using standard statistical formulas. To do this, it is necessary to specify what quantitative change is expected or hoped for in the intervention (for example, a 10% increase in breast cancer screening from 70–80% following the intervention)

Scales or scores composite summaries of existing variables intended to produce an overall score to reflect an underlying dimension (for example, six questions or items might be summed to produce an overall 'depression score')

Scaling up defined as an intervention that was demonstrated to be efficacious/effective in a small-scale study or trial and is to be expanded under real-world conditions to reach a greater proportion of the eligible population

Secular trends describe the rate of background changes in a phenomenon over a long period of time in a population (for example, national rates of smoking may be declining and obesity rates may be increasing over time)

Social mobilisation organised efforts to promote or enhance the actions and control of social groups over the **determinants** of health. This includes mobilisation of human and material resources in social action to overcome structural barriers to health, to enhance social support and to reinforce social norms conducive to health

Statistical significance a measure of the extent to which the relationship between variables, or observed results, from a study might have occurred by chance. Statistical significance is assessed after the application of appropriate statistical tests

Structured discussions a qualitative research technique, the purpose of which is to elicit information or perceptions from structured questions that are defined in advance. Structured discussions may be with individuals, as semi-structured interviews, or with groups of people, as in the conduct of focus groups

Summative evaluation different definitions of summative evaluation are available and it is sometimes used to describe the mostly quantitative impact and outcome evaluation results. A broader definition is that it considers different levels of evaluation, process and impact, and also economic evaluation, and *triangulates* data to reach a conclusion about a program's overall usefulness and **effectiveness**. It is different to *meta-evaluation*, which is a review of different evaluations to reach a summary conclusion about the net intervention effects, based on the consideration of several evaluation studies

Time-series design the set of procedures used to evaluate a health promotion intervention in which there are multiple measurements preceding intervention, followed by multiple post-intervention measurements of the outcome of interest

Triangulation the process of comparing different evaluation findings that are accumulated from a variety of sources; for example, comparing results on program **effectiveness** by examining quantitative data, and then considering if qualitative information points to the same direction and degree of effectiveness

Type 1 error where the researcher concludes that a health promotion program has produced significant outcomes (positive or negative), and when it has not (this is 'rejecting the null hypothesis when it is true')

Type 2 error where a program effect is said to be non-significant when in fact it is. A type 2 error occurs when a research project fails to reject the null hypothesis, in other words, the evaluation reported a non-significant effect of the intervention, when the true effect was that it was significant. A type 2 error may also occur when the study is underpowered, with too few people in the study to detect the effects being sought

Validity the assessment of the 'truth' of a measurement. A question, scale or test is considered valid to the extent it measures what it intended to measure. The concept of *face validity* is that experts in the field think the measure is a useful way of assessing the dimension of interest. The concept of *content validity* is that the items cover all of the potential areas of interest ('domains' of interest) expected for the measure. *Construct validity* describes the extent to which the 'construct' that is being measured in a study (for example, self-efficacy, social capital or quality of life) is actually measured by the questions or items used in a study. The usual method for identifying a construct is through statistical techniques, such as latent variable methods, exploratory or confirmatory factor analysis and internal consistency reliability, so that one can tell if the items seem to be statistically part of a single construct or dimension. This is known as *construct validation*

Variables quantitative measures that are (validly and reliably) assessed and, as the name suggests, capable of showing variation between subjects and variation in response to intervention. Variables may be single items (single questions) or summarised as composite **scales or scores**

index

Page numbers in **bold** print refer to main entries.

A

academics, xiii
acceptability, 94
'action research', 33
actions *see* health promotion actions
adaptation, evaluating, 94
adoption, 52
advocacy, 8, 10, 141
analysis of data, 33, **77–9**, 138,
    see also statistical tests
assessment of uptake, 113

B

before–after (pre–post) studies, 70–1,
    73, 96, 109, 146
behavioural epidemiology, 25, 141
best practice, identifying, 40, 137
bias, 141
    non-response, 75
    response, 84
    selection, **74–7**

C

case studies
    formative evaluation, using, 41–2,
        43–5
    immunisation, 26, 31
    physical activity promotion, 25, 30
    skin cancer prevention, 29, 32
    stages of evaluation, 30–2
    STI intervention, 27, 31
    sun protection, 28–9, 31, 97
cluster randomised controlled trials, 28,
    72, 95, 141
cohort studies, 70, 84, 141
community
    consultation with target groups,
        39–40
    impact of program over time on,
        11–12

value judgments by, xiii
comparison populations, 68–9
complex program evaluation (CPE),
    18, **89–102**, 141
    background, 89–92
    calculating cost-effectiveness, 99,
        135–6
    challenges in conducting, 97–100
    evaluation designs, 95–7
    examples in published papers, 100–1
    formative and process valuation, 92–4
    history, 91
    hypothetical example, 99–100
    planning and evaluation stages, 92
concepts, 82, 142
conclusions (interpretations), 139
confidence intervals, 78, 142
confirmatory factor analysis, 135, 150
confounding factors, 79, 142
consistency in scales and scores, 82
CONSORT criteria, 130
construct validity, 82, 135, 142
consultation with target groups,
    39–40, 142
contamination (of control groups),
    69, 142
content validity, 82, 142
context, 53–4, 55, 93, 126
control (comparison) populations, 68–9
    quasi-experimental designs, 69–72
controlled trials, 67–9
convenient sampling, 76, 148
correlates of health outcomes, 26,
    42–3, 142
cost-effectiveness, calculating, 99, **135–6**
critical appraisal of evidence, **124–7**
critical practitioners, 119, **129**
cross-sectional studies, 26, 70, 143
    response bias and, 84

D

data analysis, 33, **77–9**, 138,
    see also statistical tests

data collection, 33–4, 71, 81, 96, 101
data source triangulation, 35, 96–7, 100
delivery, 53, 55, 112
design *see* evaluation design
determinants of health, 6, 7, 9, 25–6, 43, 91, 143, *see also* intermediate health outcomes
diabetes prevention, hypothetical intervention, **131–3**
diffusion of innovation theory, 112
dissemination, 143, *see also* intervention dissemination
  compared with 'diffusion', 112
drop out, 75, 143

E

economic evaluations, **135–6**
education, to improve health literacy, 9–10
effect size, 77, 109, 143, *see also* outcome evaluation
effectiveness, 6, 19, 27, 52, 119, 143
efficacy, 18–20, 27, 52, 119, 143
engagement of stakeholders, 19, 108
environmental factors, 6, 9, 11, 32, 55, 122
epidemiology, 23
  behavioural, 25, 141
  social, 25, 141
errors, *see* biases
evaluability assessment, 41
evaluation, xiii–xiv, **11–12**, 143,
    see also research evidence; value judgments
  art and science of, **128–9**
  critical appraisal of evidence, **124–7**
  formative *see* formative evaluation
  getting evidence into policy, **123–4**
  getting evidence into practice, **119–23**
  health promotion programs, xiii
  impact, 11
  institutionalised programs, 114–16
  methods and types, **17–19**, **64–87**
  outcome *see* outcome evaluation
  planning for, **1–15**
  practical need balanced with scientific design, **19–22**
  process *see* process evaluation
  quantitative or qualitative methods, **32–5**

sampling and recruitment in, 75
stages, **22–32**
summative, 91
evaluation design, 143–4
  challenges in, 4
  choosing 'best possible', 67
  different measures for different purposes, **85–6**
  for complex programs, 95–7
  health promotion projects, **65–74**
  intervention demonstration (replication), **27–9**
  multiple *see* triangulation of information
  randomised controlled trials, 67–9, 141
  replication and dissemination, **110–14**
  typology of measures, 7
evidence *see* evaluation designs; research evidence
experimental designs, **72–4**
exploratory factor analysis, 150
exposure, 53, 54, 55
external validity, 20, 112

F

face validity, 82, 144, 150
factor analysis, 135, 150
fidelity of program delivery, 6, 54, 94, 144
flexibility, 94, 98
formative evaluation, 4, 5, 11, 23, 25, **38–48**, 137, 144
  best practice, identifying, 40, 137
  definition, 35
  examples in published papers, 43–5
  for complex program evaluation, **92–4**, 100–1, 113
  for large-scale, multi-component programs, 47
  for mass media campaigns, 47
  testing methods and materials, **38–46**

G

generalisability of results, 20, 54, 75, 108, 144
goals, 5, 144
'grey literature', 125

H

health education, 9–10
health literacy, 9–10, 66, 79, 108, 144
health practitioners, xiii, 110
health promotion actions, 7–10
health promotion outcomes, 6, 7–11,
    51, 144
  intermediate *see* intermediate health
    promotion outcomes
  intervention demonstration
    see intervention demonstration
    (replication)
  long-term, 7, 8, 117
  measurement of *see* measurements
  short-term, 5, 8
health promotion programs
  assessing effects of *see* impact
    evaluation; outcome evaluation
  critical appraisal checklist, **136–140**
  evaluation of, **64–87**
  getting evidence into policy, **123–4**
  getting evidence into practice, **119–23**
  goals and objectives, 1, 2, 5, 19
  individual, appraisal of, 137–9
  planning and evaluation cycle, 2, 13
  population-level, 89–90
  post-intervention appraisal,
    139–40
  single-component, moving to
    complex program evaluation,
    89–90
health service monitoring, 115–16
healthy environments, 7–10, 79
healthy lifestyle, 7, 8, 10, 101
HIV health promotion program,
    7, 9–10, 44, 57, 59, 90, 121

I

immunisation case study, 26, 31
impact, 19
impact evaluation, 11, 26–7,
    39, 51, 87, 92, 131, 144,
    see also outcome evaluation
  assessing program effects, 39
  definition, 35
  for complex programs, 95, 100–1
  identifying target groups, 66
  stages in assessing significance, 105–7
implementation of programs

see program implementation
indicators *see* evaluation designs;
    measurements; measures and
    indicators
influence, 6, 8
innovation diffusion theory, 112
innovation testing, 24, **26–7**, 31
institutionalisation, **104–6**, 144, *see also*
    intervention dissemination
  evaluation methods for, **114–16**
  monitoring, 114–15
  post-intervention appraisal, 140
intermediate health outcomes, 7–11,
    144, 145
  determinants of health, 7, 91
  impact evaluation, 11
  measurement of, 79
internal consistency, 82, 145, *see also*
    consistency in scales and scores
internal consistency, 145
internal validity, 20
interpretation of results, 139
inter-rater reliability, 81, 86, 134, 148
intervention demonstration
    (replication), 24, **27–9**, 31, 104–6,
    see also health promotion outcomes
  evaluation methods, **107–11**
intervention dissemination, 23, 24, **29**,
    32, 104–7
  evaluation methods, **111–14**
  examples in published papers, 110–11
  post-intervention appraisal, 139
intervention mapping, 4, 13, 14, 41,
    46, 51
interventions *see* health promotion
    programs

K

knowledge translation *see* research
    translation

L

logic models, 4, 13, **14–15**, 41, 46,
    51, 145
  for complex program evaluation,
    99–100
  school canteen improvement, 14–15
long-term health promotion outcomes,
    7, 8, 145

M

maturation of cohorts, 84
measurement
    across different stages of evaluation,
        85–6
    bias, 80–1, 141
    complex programs, of, 96
    different measures for different
        purposes, **85–6**
    errors, 75, 80–1
    health promotion outcomes,
        79–87, 138
    issues that can influence results, 84
    purpose of, **82–5**
    statistical tests *see* statistical tests
    reliability and validity, 80–2, 133–5
measures and indicators, 80, 145
media campaigns, 45, 47, 90
mediators, theoretical, 60, 133
meta-analysis, 126, 127, 137, 145
methods
    evaluation, of, **17–19**, **64–87**
    testing *see* formative evaluation
mobilisation of resources *see* resource
        mobilisation
monitoring
    health service delivery, 115–16
    institutionalisation, 114
multiple-agency partnership
        program, 18

N

non-observable phenomena, 32,
        145, 146
non-response bias, 75, 146
numeric data, 33

O

objectives, 5, 146
observable phenomena, 32, 79, 146
observations *see* qualitative methods
organisational practices, 8, 9
outcome evaluation, 23, 26–7, **35**, 36,
        39, 41, 131, 146, *see also* impact
        evaluation
outcomes, **7–11**
    determinants of health *see* health
        promotion outcomes
    impact measures, 11–12
    intermediate *see* intermediate
        health outcomes
    long-term *see* health promotion
        outcomes
    short-term *see* health promotion
        outcomes
    theoretical distribution over time, 12

P

participation (recruitment), 53, 55, 66
participatory planning (consultation),
        14, 40, 146
physical activity promotion, 25, 30, 59
pilot testing, 146
    intervention materials, 26, 40–1, 42,
        46
planning and evaluation cycle, 2, 13
planning for evaluation, **1–15**
policy change, 123–4
policy-makers, xiii, 19, 28, 29, 47, 95,
        96, 108, 111, 119, 121, 123, 129
'political engagement', 113
population-level health promotion,
        89–90, 105–6
population surveillance, 96–7, 115
post-intervention appraisal, 139–40
practical need, balanced with scientific
        design, **19–22**
practitioner perspectives, xiii, 21–2, 55
pre-experimental designs, 69, 74
pre–post (before–after) studies, 70–1,
        73, 96, 109, 146
prevalence, 3, 25, 146
preventive health services, effective, 7
problem definition, **3–4**, 24, **25**, 30, 137
process evaluation, 6, 26, 38, 46,
        51–61, 137, 146, *see also* program
        implementation
    assessing implementation, 23, **51–4**
    definition, 35
    examples in published papers, 57–9
    for complex program evaluation,
        92–4, 100–1
    institutionalisation phase, 115
    methods for conducting, **54–7**
    practical tasks in, 55
    replication stage, 110
program fidelity, 6, 53, 94
program implementation, **5–6**, 85, 96,

99, 109, 110, *see also* intervention demonstration (replication); intervention dissemination; process evaluation
practitioner perspectives, 21
program monitoring, **30**, 32, 53
program plans, 3–5, 147
using formative evaluation, 41
project or intervention, 147
public health programs, 17, 24, 104
complex, 19, 90–2, 141
identifying target group, 66
public policy, 9

Q

qualitative methods, **32–5**, 56, 73, 91, 147
'quality' assessment, 30
quantitative methods, **32–5**, 54, 57, 74, 98, 79, 95, 147
quasi-experimental designs, **69–72**, 73–4, 95, 141, 147

R

random sampling, 75, 75, 147
randomised controlled trials (RCTs), 67, 141, 147
CONSORT criteria for, 130
examples of, 72–4
for complex programs, 95
reach, 23, 52, 54, 89, 93, 139, 147
reactive practice, 121
'real-world' conditions *see* effectiveness; process evaluation
recruitment, 75, *see also* sampling techniques
relevance, 19
reliability (reproducibility), **83**, 148
of measurement, 80–3, 133–5
self-confidence example, 60, 81, 83
'repeatability' of measurement, 86, 133
repetition, 108
replication, 28, **107–11**, 148, *see also* intervention demonstration (replication)
evaluation methods, 109–11
examples in published papers, 110–11
post-intervention appraisal, 139

representativeness, 148
reproducibility *see* reliability
research design *see* evaluation design
research evidence *see also* evaluation; scientific design
critical appraisal of evidence, **124–7**
getting it into policy, **123–4**
getting it into practice, **119–23**
value judgments, xiii
research synthesis, 124
research translation, 107–8
resource assessments, 5
resource mobilisation, 2, 9, *see also* engagement of stakeholders
response bias, 84
responsiveness, 82, 83, 120–1, 148
retention of subjects, 75, 146

S

sample, 148
sample size, 85, 148
calculation, 77
type 2 errors, 81, 84, 149
sampling techniques, **75–7**, 130, 138
satisfaction and usage, 53
satisfaction surveys, 54
scales (measurements), 82, 148
scaling up, 23, 104, 106–8, 112, 113, 148
school canteen improvement, 14–15
scientific design *see also* experimental designs; quantitative methods; research evidence
balanced with practical need, **19–22**
building evidence for public health programs, 64
scientific reviews, 40
scores (measurements), 82, 148
secular trends, 78, 148–9
selection bias, **74–7**, 138, 141
minimising, 75
self-confidence example, 60, 81, 83
sensitisation to issues, 84
sensitivity to change, 82
short-term health promotion outcomes, 5, 8
significance (statistical testing), 21, 33, 68, **77–9**, 105–7, 149

single-component interventions
  moving to complex program
  evaluation, 89–90
  reaching whole populations, 90
smoking prevention programs, 10
  case study, 28–9, 31
  process evaluation of, 60
snowball sampling, 76, 148
social action and influence, 9
social epidemiology, 25
social health outcomes, 8
social mobilisation, 8, **9–10**, 79, 149
socio-ecological framework, 4
'soft' research, 34
solution generation, 2, 24, **25–6**, 31
stages of evaluation, **22–32**
  measurement across, 85–6
stakeholders, engagement of, 19, 108
statistical methods, **77–8**
statistical significance, 21, 33, 68, **77–9**,
  105–7, 149
statistical tests, **77–8**, *see also* data
  analysis; measurements
  example, hypothetical diabetes
    prevention, **131–3**
  quantitative method, 33
  reliability and validity, 80–2, 133–5
stepped-wedge design, 68, 72, 74, 95
STI intervention case study, 27, 31
structured discussions, 33, 149
study design *see* evaluation design
study samples *see* sampling
  techniques
subject retention, 75, 146
summative evaluation, 91, 97, 149
sun protection case study, 28–9, 31, 97

sustainability, 94
systematic reviews, 40, 126–7
systems approaches, 91, 113

T
target groups
  consultation with, 39–40
  identification of, 66–7
test–re-test procedures, 81, 86
testing methods and materials
  see formative evaluation
time-series designs, 70–1, 83, 149
TREND statement, **136**
triangulation of information,
  35, 96–7, 100, 149
type 1 errors, 81, 84, 149
type 2 errors, 81, 84, 149

U
uptake, 113
'usual care', 68
utilisation, 52

V
validity, 80–2, 133–5, 150
  of measurement, 80–2, 133–5
value judgments, xiii, *see also* evaluation
  variables
variables, 27, 150

W
weight-loss, hypothetical intervention,
  131–3

Y
youth smoking, case study, 28–9, 31